Parsifal's Journal

A Compendium of The Knowledge Of Everything

Parsifal's Journal

A Compendium of The Knowledge Of Everything

Anthony Wakefield Hill

ATHENA PRESS
LONDON

ISBN 978 1 84748 565 6

First published 2009 by
ATHENA PRESS
Queen's House, 2 Holly Road
Twickenham TW1 4EG
United Kingdom

Printed for Athena Press

<u>Forthcoming Titles by Anthony Wakefield Hill 2009</u>

The One and the Many – The Basis of all Knowledge

The Knowledge of Everything – The Actuality of all Knowledge

The Revolutionising of Medical Procedure – Physical and Mental

Parsifal's Journal – Issues 2, 3 & 4

Introduction

Parsifal's Journal is a four-monthly compendium of literary and intellectual essays on every subject known to man, leavened by a serial account of the singular life of Parsifal himself.

This first volume of the journal is in the form of a manifesto from the secure ward of a psychiatric hospital, where our hero has been forcibly detained, through no fault of his own, and without having offered any resistance to his arrest. The circumstances of Parsifal's arrest are particularly obscure, and shrouded in the mysteries of the unfathomable psychiatric mentality – though not unfathomable to Parsifal himself, who understands the medical profession only too well, as will become clear in the course of this collection of writings.

It has become necessary for this divinely-originated philosopher to publish his own magazine because of the incomprehensible refusal of the Spectator, over the last five years to publish any of his weekly contributions, and also because of the equally mulish reluctance on the part of the Sunday Telegraph, and other publications, to comply with this request.

I wish to make it clear that my references to 'Venus' throughout this magazine, in no way involve a particular person, but only a composite Woman – in particular, the One Woman of all mens' imagination.

In view of the fact that my incarceration in this hospital is to be of an 'indeterminable length', I am forced to make a desperate appeal for help, to all open-minded and intelligent people – of whom there are a great few out there. I am not asking for you to support any claim that I am Christ; I am merely asking you to support my pleas for freedom from drugs and hospitalisation, and from further interference from psychiatry. I have never harmed anyone in my life and the claim that I 'might be a danger to myself' is too ludicrous to entertain. If I like to think I am Jesus, is it a crime? Is it an offence to anything but psychiatry's conceited sense of its own propriety? Isn't this a free country?

I have never even claimed <u>to a member of the public</u> that I am Jesus Christ – so uninterested am I in any kudos occurring from it. <u>To whom</u> can it cause any harm? – And how much good <u>might</u> it do?

You will see from my many books, just what good I can do.

I ask some of those who knew me, forty-five years ago, to stand up for me, in my very dire straits. It would be useful to have the testimonies of the two doctors who examined me, approximately thirty years ago, one of whom was a Dutch psychoanalyst (with an unpronounceable name) and the other was an English psychologist in a hospital in North London; they were professionally connected.

Contents

I hereby declare that I am the Lord of the Universe, come to earth to kill your ego, and to instruct you in the ways of thinking.

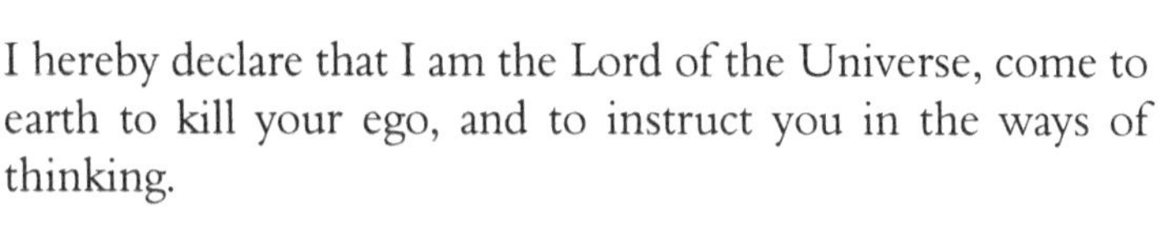

After sixty years as the world's arsehole, I am at last resurrected.

I require you to prosecute me.

Letter to the Editor of the Sunday Telegraph and of the Spectator

Sir,

This letter is an extension of the one I sent you exactly a fortnight ago, in which I asked you to publish my articles on a regular basis. I partly retract this request in favour of a perhaps less regular publication, whereby you would not have to actually employ me – if that is a barrier to my acceptance. I am perfectly prepared to write without being paid, and certainly not as an actual columnist – if again that is a barrier – but on the condition that my articles are indeed published, as and when I write them. I therefore see no reason why they should not be accepted.

You have failed to reply to me – a gross discourtesy and an omission which can only be regarded as a calculated insult. Nor have you featured such articles as I have already sent you; if your minions have not passed them on to you, by God I'll have their bloody balls for cocktail onions.

On no grounds can these articles be dismissed as 'unsuitable' – and thanks to you personally they will now be well and truly out of date. I understood that editors did not shirk controversy or hard-hitting truth; surely that is what newspapers are about? 'The public don't want to read it', you protest: <u>don't give</u> the public what it wants to read. Journalists pride themselves on <u>leading</u> public opinion – or so I thought; newspaper editors are not noted for their courage, however – despite their boasts about being avant garde and in the forefront of public debate…

You produce a gutless, lukewarm and sycophantic rag – and before you toss this aside, have a thought for us who dare to speak the truth and <u>need</u> a platform – not for our good but for the good of the nation, whose interests <u>you</u> should have at heart. Your concern with the sensibilities of the public over what needs to be heard does you and your paper no credit.

Just in case you are trying to inform me I am 'Jesus Christ', I should point out that I am already in possession of the facts, and it is a decision only I can take in any case.

If you are worried about being sued – don't be; I am quite prepared to go to court on my own behalf.

If, alternatively, you are miffed about my trying to get onto the Spectator and Sunday Telegraph at the same time, you needn't be; whichever of you turns up trumps will have the privilege of my contributions.

After all this, if you still refuse to recognize the overwhelming importance, the crucial nature – <u>vital</u> nature – of these essays for the citizens of this country, then you are an absolute, malicious twerp. If you had any morals, any integrity – any spunk – you would not hesitate to publish this work. And if you do not, it will be the most shameful injustice imaginable – but I expect that injured ego and spite will persuade you to consign me to oblivion – won't it?

I think I am at least entitled to a reply, by way of explanation.

P.S. In the unlikely event that you <u>are</u> trying to convince me I am Jesus Christ, how can I be expected to guess that without a statement from someone? Stony silence does not convey anything; let yourself be the first person in the last forty years who has been forthcoming to me.

<u>Unreplied to</u>

Civilization And The Aftermath Of Slavery

Enough of this recent nonsense about the slave-trade. Is the British government going to be railroaded by some opportunistic Africans over something that happened nearly two-hundred years ago? No, it isn't true that modern-day attitudes originated with slavery: racism has been inherent in every race since time began – including African races. African tribes have enslaved other African peoples for thousands of years, and, almost to this day, the Arab people of North Africa and elsewhere have enslaved the Negroes of the south.

Were not the British forced into slavery by the Romans? Are we to hold the present-day Italians responsible for that? – to demand that they apologise? Every conquering race in history has subjected others to bondage. And let it not be forgotten: it was the British who put a stop to the slave-trade. I, for one, am fed up with this culture of Britain-bashing.

———————

Before I continue, a short note on racism:

The 'evil of racism in our society' is due to one thing: the white man's fear of the natural emotions <u>in himself</u>, particularly in our Western society where the instincts are repressed; which results in the projection of our own forbidden emotions onto the unfortunate black man, who thus represents all that we hate within ourselves.

———————

Africa is ablaze – with primordial horror and insatiable blood-lust. We in the cosseted security of Britain's privileged Civilization find it hard to envisage the unbridled savagery of these primitive races. Fratricide, mutual slaughter and collective insanity are endemic across the continent, Africans being distinctly animal in nature; so little advanced are they up the evolutionary ladder that they still remain in the animal kingdom, daily exhibiting the rampant law of the jungle: primitivism at its naked worst.

In this steaming cauldron of violence, vicious hatred is waiting constantly to be sparked off; and when the excuse comes, primeval madness is unleashed. Brother turns on brother, women and children are butchered, innocents are macheted to death. Very near the surface lurks the primordial Beast, never having been tamed, never civilized, waiting to be released by the demon of unconscious instinct. We are witnessing the other face of primitivism – the true one? This rabid continent is far from innocent.

This frightful maw of primitive existence is infested with crocodile and snake-ridden men and women turning on each other and hacking, gouging and bludgeoning themselves into the bloody morass surrounding them – which sucks them ever further into its ghastly womb. The matrix of creation proves to be a diabolical hell- hole, where <u>raw energy</u> devours everything that falls into it – truly the 'black hole' of Hawking's nightmarish vision, translated from physical into mental terms.

The only way out of this hole, this festering pit, is by <u>individuality</u>; i.e. Civilization, to which Africa has yet to aspire. Individuality alone is capable of lifting man out of chaos, by virtue of its co-respondent, consciousness – as yet alien to the jungle-bound peasant. Unliberated Africans must look to their feminine – <u>the woman within</u>; the only arbiter of salvation. Macho youths and men, at present deluded and misled by the masculine ego, can only be rescued by their better half: womanly consciousness. Awake, o'ye who would come out of Africa!

Even in the primeval slime, ego exists, unacknowledged, unconscious to mankind in general; take heed of this devilish predator beneath the awareness of all of us.

Despite all, hope yet lives in Africa, in this erstwhile cradle of innocence – the obverse side of instinct. Good and evil never held potentially greater sway than in the crucible of this continent; though the <u>conflict</u> between the two has never yet been felt – lying dormant in the recesses of Unity – with a salutary dose of consciousness this latent cross could indeed save what is at present a truly primitive race. Innocents of Africa, I salute you!

The question of 'aids' arises here, being the indirect result of Britain's civilizing influence. When the primitive mentality comes into contact with civilization, all hell breaks loose; innocence goes out of the door, and all varieties of perversion take place. It seems that the primitive is easily seduced by 'civilized' – in this case, illicit – sexuality; Western culture has nothing to be proud of here.

Unfortunately, no-one, whether in Africa or Europe, seems ashamed of this disease, which is brought about by nothing less than promiscuity – the most wanton and degrading abandonment of all natural instinct and self-respect. The African seems particularly susceptible to this, and it is no wonder that certain of us observers are appalled, and seek to condemn it; aids <u>should</u> be discriminated against; it rightly bears a stigma. These pariahs, whether African or European, are actually condoned by the Church, the government and all seemingly respectable institutions – even attaining recognition as saints and 'unfortunate victims' of some perfectly understandable, even innocent injustice. But telling this to the intellectual establishment is like pissing in the wind.

Africa's governmental institutions are riddled with incompetence at all levels; bribery and corruption and downright economic chaos are rife. You may claim the right to self-government, but you <u>can't</u> govern yourselves; look at the mess you've made of it. And <u>don't</u> put it down to 'post-colonialism'; there is a gross lack of intelligence involved, plus a cultural void.

The 'right to govern yourselves' is <u>not</u> self-evident. Nobody has the <u>right</u> to do anything. You would be lucky if God granted you the right to breathe, which is his option to give and his alone; he did not accompany it with any further obligation on his part. Human existence is a <u>gift</u>, not bestowing the privilege to demand anything.

God does not say you have a right to self-government; such rights as you have are made <u>by</u> man <u>for</u> man, and as such are far from self- evident. If you want self-government, you have to earn it – to show that you are capable of it. You may have the man-made right to make your own mistakes, but not at the expense of human life and civilized values. 'Europe killed six million Jews', you say, but in fact Germany killed them, and not any other European state; for which Germany was ostracized and duly punished. Britain went to war partly to <u>save</u> the Jews; and two world-wars were forced on us <u>by</u> Germany. We in Europe have, at least, a veneer of civilization.

Human life is the only right anyone has – courtesy of God; beyond that, existence is a free-for-all, with the order of battle being 'first come, first served'.

When the white man can be himself, he will be black;

When the black man can see himself, he will be white.

Global Warming

Why all this fuss about global warming? It is my intention to prove that not only is all this hype based on irrational hysteria, but that also the actual causes of global warming have been falsely assessed by science.

There is no reason to believe, apart from biased assertions, that this phenomenon has any other origin than the natural cycle of the earth itself. It is hard to accredit the emotional fervour with which this is denied to anything other than wilful contrariness. The facts speak for themselves.

The blind insistence on the part of scientists, intellectuals and politicians that this crisis – if indeed it is a crisis – is due to man's failure to control pollution, is demonstrable nonsense. It is generally accepted, and maintained by the scientists themselves, that science has actually proved man-made emissions to be the cause of global warming. It is a fact also that many other scientists have proved the opposite. The pro-emissions lobby has not advanced one single item of actual proof for their belief. They have <u>assumed</u> their theories from undoubted evidence; but it is only evidence – that evidence being that carbon emissions are indeed penetrating the upper, or lower atmosphere and may even be contributing to global warming. In comparison to the earth's own influence however, these factors are negligible and even if the proposed measures to counteract the situation were put into place they would be but a drop in the ocean. How can man prevail against the overwhelming might of the earth's own power? In fact we cannot do anything about it. We may take avoiding action, such as building flood-barriers but no-one can stop the accumulating force of the planet's direction.

The driving force of global climatic change comes from inside the earth, possibly influenced also from space, i.e. from the planets or the sun. Throughout the earth's history, climate change has regularly come about, it did not start a mere ten years ago. Is there any reason to think that in the twenty-first century it should no longer be applicable? The fact that evolution has lately resulted in civilization – which has apparently blinded science to reality – does not mean that the earth's habits have changed – and as I have said, there are many among the body of scientists who have actually proved that this is so, which of course has been ignored by those less intelligent. Science doesn't like its theories to be disproved.

If asked why I maintain that global warming is caused by natural occurrences, I answer that there is <u>no</u> reason to believe otherwise and <u>every</u> reason to believe that it is due to the earth's natural assertion of its regular climatic cycle. In any case, global warming is not an irreversible process, since, ten thousand years from now, the polar regions will probably revert to ice due to <u>global freezing</u>, as has always been the case with natural climate change. However, whilst the polar regions were becoming colder, other parts of the world were becoming distinctly hotter. If Polar regions are becoming tropical swamps, I do not see why other areas would not become subject to severe cold as in the past – or has this habitual occurrence suddenly died out to support sciences' claims?

England's last great warm up – and not only England's – starting say seven or eight thousand years ago – took place either when the arctic was an icy waste – which it largely still is – or whilst it was freezing over after its last warm period.

Therefore it seems that <u>internal</u> climate change and <u>universal</u> climate change <u>took place independently and at the same time</u> though due no doubt to the same driving force. Even if the Arctic has been frozen over for perhaps millions of years, <u>internal</u> climate change has been taking place independently and more frequently. The two may not coincide at all times, because the planet as a whole evidently takes longer to tick over under certain conditions, for which reason alone the accepted view of climate change is flawed, it not being an exclusively universal phenomenon.

If therefore internal climate fluctuation takes place independently of global climate fluctuation, heating up and cooling down autonomously, it is not hard to see that such an event involving cooler temperatures may be occurring now – unusually severe temperatures in Europe and Russia recently providing further evidence. The fact that this has gone unremarked shows how blinkered science is by its own preoccupations; if indeed it has been noticed, its significance has nevertheless been ignored. This is not just a mistake, but a symptom of a deep seated illness within the human psyche.

Global warming as with global freezing, is not a universal process, both climatic conditions taking place simultaneously. Therefore I think it highly likely that we will see coinciding planetary heating and planetary cooling. The severe winters seen over the last several years in various parts of the world, are, if acknowledged at all, regarded as a 'blip'. But the fact that they are so widespread, and so extreme, must indicate something more permanent – and more significant.

The actual cause of all these climate-change, and other, scares is the inability of science to think. Their so-called reasons are actually a knee jerk reaction – irrational and scatty cogitation. This panic-driven thinking – which isn't thinking at all – actually panics us into even more ill considered assessments of the original situation, which becomes more obscured with the ever mounting myopia of our experts – particularly with the inflexible egotism lying behind the beliefs of scientists.

If you do not accept this account, I ask you to look for once behind the scenes, to the reality driving most predictions – which would require thought if science thought at all. All science does is to observe, such experiments as it may perform being based on false assumptions from the very start.

Scientists do not know what lies beneath physical appearances; therefore any judgments they may make are based entirely on what is observed above the surface, which, obviously, is bound to mislead the uninformed investigator.

Thinking according to science, therefore, has a very shaky basis. Within their discipline researchers are no doubt exactly right; but when it comes to the very much larger picture, science is blind.

In order to experiment on something, you first of all have to know whether it exists; and, to cut a long story short, no phenomenon whatever, in the physical world, actually has any objective existence. Mathematics itself is based on the preliminary assumption that two and two make four, whereas, in the real world, they make five, six, or even seven. Lacking any insight, then, into the reality behind climate change, our researchers presume to teach the rest of us that the upper atmosphere is pissing on us, on the basis that the ozone layer is <u>presumed</u> to exhibit a reaction to carbon emissions. The fact that the ozone layer exists, and the fact that the carbon emissions exist, is enough to convince the scientist that there is a connection between the two, but, actually, whatever reaction is occurring to the ozone layer could equally well be caused by a large variety of things.

Two and two <u>may</u> equal four, but there are many possibilities interposing themselves <u>between</u> these two numbers, so confounding any attempt to make a hard-and-fast calculation.

Even if there is evidence of carbon emissions within the ozone layer, this does not prove that carbon emissions are the cause of the widening hole; still less does it prove that greenhouse gases are responsible for global warming.

There is a world of infinite possibility between two and four.

Dear Archbishop

I enclose a letter concerning the recent sharia debacle, in which I am entirely on your side; do take the trouble to read it.

Whatever disparaging remarks I make about the clergy, I exempt you from them, considering you a brave, intelligent and honest man. The letter really speaks for itself, but 1 hope you are intelligent enough to embrace the novel idea of a prophet in your midst.

Highly unlikely as it might seem, I am forced, much against my retiring inclination, to declare myself; I do not know whether you have heard of me – you would only have been a boy when I came into prominence forty five years ago, having been pronounced the 'prophet of the age' by a group of psychoanalysts who rescued me from obscurity – not to say condemnation as a madman (a diagnosis, I may say, which I personally fully endorsed).

If at this point you tear up this letter in disgust, I shall fully understand; but I would make the plea that I am in dire need of an ally in my mission, which is in acute danger of being scuppered by the ignorant reactions of the intellectual establishment, refusing, as they do, to publish my ideas under any circumstances. Any excuse will do as long as I am muzzled like a rabid dog. I am not asking you to proclaim who I am, or even to believe who I am, but simply to afford me the opportunity to communicate with you on a more or less regular basis.

I know you to be a forward looking man – re: your views on homosexuality, Sharia law, etc – and I rather expect that you will not dismiss me out of hand; though I have given you no proof of my identity – and let me for the moment remain nameless – let me just say it is obvious that hard headed psychoanalysts do not acclaim someone as a prophet without very good reason, and if, as I hope, you are acquainted with C.G. Jung's writings (being a competent intellectual yourself, with presumably an enquiring mind) you may be aware of the predicted advent of a person like myself.

Please do not write me off as a crank – at least until you have read some examples of my work – which, 'heretical' as it may be in tone, is actually designed to instruct human kind in the true ways of the Lord. Apocalyptic though my vision may be, it comes at a time in the affairs of the world when such a thing would be appropriate, and, despite its revolutionary nature, eligible for acceptance by all who possess an open mind and an instinctive awareness of what Christianity means for the modern world.

Christ himself, though even he was not a fully conscious being, indicated that this revelation was to come, and I, unfortunately for myself, have been chosen for the mouthpiece of the Voice of the very pregnant Silence. I say 'unfortunately' because owing to my bounteous love for this planet and all its inhabitants, I will actually seek to endure an unprecedentedly horrible death – far worse than crucifixion.

But only through this death will the world be reconciled to itself, at the same time being awakened to the true meaning of The Eternal Life. For I bear witness that Heaven exists on earth, <u>or will do when man becomes conscious of it.</u> I may be rating your intelligence too high, and in any case I wouldn't blame you for tearing this up, but I entreat you to listen to me – not for my sake but for that of both yours, and my, long suffering devotees, to whom this mission is long overdue – two thousand years almost exactly.

At any rate please reply to me, upon receipt of which I will send you a treatise on the twenty-first century reality of life and death, specifically dealing with the combination of Reincarnation and the One Life within the 'Eternal Life'; as promised by Jesus so long ago.

As the reconciling agent between East and West, I hope to have the opportunity to put my case before you, and the honour to be your friend.

Yours sincerely

Anthony Wakefield Hill

The Sharia Debacle

Archbishop Williams is a beleaguered and unjustifiably vilified man. In fact the claim by some of his Bishops that this is a case of public hysteria, and knee jerk reaction on the part of the press, is quite correct. It is a most unintelligent, misinformed and vindictive response. Obviously – it goes without saying – the Archbishop would not advocate flogging or beheading or familial murder; such a suggestion is ludicrous.

If Sharia law is complicated, if British law is complicated, if a combination of the two is complicated, surely an accommodation on both sides is possible? Is it beyond the power of the judiciary to work out a few reasonable caveats for exceptional cases?

I do not see the problem; it is not the Very Reverend Williams who is naive, but the British public. The real problem is the blinkered, unthinking and malicious reflexes on the part of society as a whole. Humankind constantly demonstrates its automaton nature in cases such as this, making blindly assumptive, assertive and totally illogical declarations against innocent people. It hounds out anyone who goes against the grain – not rationally but like a zombie performing in its sleep. Such is the collective identity that it can not <u>see</u>, being wrapped in insupportable unconsciousness for most of its supposedly waking life.

In the human psyche, thought does not exist, consisting rather, of reactive instinct and emotional impulse, which produces constant imaginary slights, irrational fears and intolerant prejudices. Its robotic nature does not allow it to see beyond its nose; by extension, the scientific mentality in particular exhibits this trait, informing and coercing the rest of humanity in this disastrous lack of perception. In the physical world, science rules all, contaminating everything with its material touch, not deigning to acknowledge the vast reaches of true intelligence lying beyond it. Science is us, science we are.

The fear, on the part of Muslim women, that Sharia law, if pursued in Britain, would lead to fratricide is groundless because any sensible judge would rule against it – assuming it ever got onto the statute books.

Why should Muslims not have special consideration as far as religious sensibilities go? As long as these do not actually conflict with an enlightened view of world religion as a whole – including Christianity- I do not see why there should be any question; surely the judiciary can apply the tenets of good and evil in an impartial manner, wherever the accused may come from? These things will have to be judged on their merits; the legal system will simply have to be made more flexible – as it is all the time. As guests in our country, all foreigners should be treated with due respect for their national and racial customs. They must respect our laws, we must respect theirs: a mutual toleration society.

Two hundred years ago in Britain, a man would probably have been hanged for murder whatever his reasons and probably regardless of his innocence. Nowadays we are more tolerant and intelligent – or so I would hope – and we would take into account his motives vis-à-vis his mental state, his marital circumstances, etc. To take one case in point, I am unable to understand why there has never been a provision for the 'crime passionel' in this country, its introduction being long overdue.

At present we hang a man merely for the <u>act</u> of murder; as long as the crime is not cold-bloodedly planned, I consider that anyone has a perfect right to kill his wife's seducer. This would not lead to mayhem – why should it? – and in fact it would introduce some much needed natural justice to an outmoded and unfair legal system. It does not give carte blanche to every would-be criminal to commit murder indiscriminately.

'Thou shalt not kill' is of course the stumbling block – according to Moses and to some antiquated clerical relics. But Moses was not a notably enlightened individual, and his authoritarian religious doctrine is not relevant, for the most part, in a modern, more open, secular world. Islam, by the way is particularly open to the same criticism, Muslim clerics, along with their reactionary Christian counterparts, being locked in an antediluvian time warp.

Unfortunately, in a contemporary society, laying down the law, particularly one introduced hundreds if not thousands of years ago, smells of ecclesiastical oppression in the worse tradition of medieval bigotry.

<u>To be an individual – the much vaunted goal of all religious, philosophical and political tradition, one must think for oneself – otherwise, by definition, no individuality.</u>

Thinking for oneself is absolutely essential if one is to attain a unique and independent consciousness, so necessary to a forward looking, and successful, society; this can not be too strongly stressed. This is what God put us on earth for: not to be pontificated to by a collection of backward looking old farts.

I mention the 'crime passionel' as an example of the one free-thinking attitude in the Muslim penal code – all credit to them for that – which, above all Islamic laws, demonstrates the Rightness and necessity for incorporating this into the British legal system. Need I also cite the French law? Who says that British Justice is the best in the world? It certainly won't be if it shows itself incapable of adaptability and sheer commonsense.

The present public furore is exacerbated by the inflammatory, wild and totally unconsidered accusations thrown about by myopic politicians and clergymen, and confused even further by naive and over-sensitive remarks from the Muslims themselves, who seem to think there is a conspiracy against them.

Who in fact is flouting British law? – which seems to be one of the main objections. The Muslim community has stated repeatedly and quite categorically that Britain's laws must remain 'paramount'. No-one is demanding an abdication on our part, but merely some comparatively minor concessions.

Why all this hysteria? Apart from the obvious and disgraceful lack of consideration, or forethought, what is the underlying reason?

Can the public not see, as I said, what is right in front of their nose? The facts are there, <u>as everyone actually knows</u>. Whence comes this wilful evasion of the truth? – from downright bloody-minded determination not to have any truck with the Muslims, under any circumstances. What happened to civil rights? To fairness for all? You may think that we are very fair in Britain: but are we? Where is our famous tolerance? And if the Archbishop gets up and utters an <u>unpopular</u> view, one which dares to challenge <u>accepted values</u>, then down comes the hatchet, and the poor man is condemned, in true medieval style, as a heretic – for defending freedom! Impartial justice! – Recognition of our neighbour's rights! – What a fiasco! What a schizophrenic mentality!

But then, again, what would you expect of the human condition? – a schizoid, self contradictory, vindictive psychosis. A mass psychosis akin to Germany's in relation to the Jews; in this case the scapegoat for the country's ills is not a victimized community but <u>one man</u>. And in case you think I am exaggerating, think on. What is it that drives humanity? It is a collective syndrome compounded of fear, malice and guilt – the guilt of men and women who, actually, unconsciously realize their wretchedness, their fecklessness, their own abysmal cowardice. No-one can bear to think he is a coward – <u>what would the others say?</u> So you look for a victim to project your fears onto.

This is a besetting and abiding preoccupation within man: I have observed it. So it ever was, so it will always be.

Fear, malice, cowardice – surmounted by Ego; an ego which says 'I cannot bear the truth, to think that I am nothing but a spineless little twerp'.

Unfortunately, the final reality of all of us. And only by recognizing this do we have any hope.

31/03/08

Re: a letter sent 21/02/08 but not dated

Your Ref: SL+1/60065

To The Archbishops' secretary:

It is five weeks since I wrote my <u>first</u> letter to the Archbishop; I wrote a <u>second</u> letter ten days later, <u>in which I asked you to personally hand my letters to the Archbishop and make sure he read them</u>.

I have had no reply to any of my letters (the first one containing two parts). The most charitable inference is that they have been lost, in which case you must be a bungling idiot. It is no excuse to say you were overwhelmed with letters – or that you and the Archbishop are too busy to bother with mine. I, too, am a busy man, and I don't expect to be relegated to the ranks of the ordinary citizen, particularly when my (original) letters were of the utmost importance.

I therefore enclose my <u>two</u> original letters again. And as I have a certain authority in this country, it would be most inadvisable for you to suppress this communication, as I will make the most almighty stink.

Dear Archbishop:

Yes, I am addressing you, the Archbishop. I insist that you read the preceding page, because it is very relevant, especially considering the incompetence of your secretary. And if he is not responsible for the absence of any reply to my two letters, sent five weeks ago, I must assume that you personally are to blame.

You have cavalierly ignored my communications, and have evidently seen fit to dismiss me personally as a 'crank'. I would have thought it common politeness to reply to my letter – notwithstanding your 'busyness' – but especially to one so vital in nature, one so obviously in need of a response. I am not asking you to believe in me – that would be too much to expect. I am merely asking you to read my dissertation on 'Life and Death' – a seminal essay I might add – which I have offered you but which you have spurned out of hand. It couldn't possibly be worth reading, could it? – your 'intellectual powers' are far above it…

I enclose copies of my <u>two</u> letters which are not primarily to do with the 'Sharia Debate'. And in case your secretary has destroyed the covering letter, I warn you both there will be hell to pay.

Anthony Wakefield Hill (A name well known among the cognoscenti)

In the light of your obvious intolerance of any unconventional approach to the Christian religion, let me point out that the Day of the Apocalypse is now at hand, and that all backward-looking priests, as a consequence, will find themselves blackballed by the Lord above, who, as the author of the book 'Revelations' did reveal this very event, or series of events. Reactionary views will not find favour in this modern world, specifically promulgated in the prescience of the Almighty. All hair-shirted and be-mitred wonders will be shunted off to the sidelines, awaiting superannuation; Christ has no time for them.

As I expected, you are the kind of self satisfied, bearded freak who would look down even on his own Messiah – prevented from recognizing him by your own massive ego; the prime disqualification, as it happens, for a man of the church. In view of the fact that you are the head of the Church of England, I do not hold out much hope for your congregation, the situation being that of a monkey in charge of the organ.

And, when I am finally recognized – which won't be far off – don't come crawling to me with unctuous protestations of remorse – because I shall reject you. If I don't get a reply from you, I will personally set fire to that bloody beard of yours.

P.S. As far as you are concerned Mr Secretary, if you fail to pass on this missive I will ensure that the morning visit to the thunderbox meets with disaster, and that you pass the rest of the day nursing a very tender arse.

Public Sector Pay

The police are a 'special case'? Balderdash. What is special about them? The usual plea is: 'We put our lives at risk' – so do many people. What about the firemen, the coastguard, the mountain rescue services; the army, the navy, the air force, the intelligence services. Do you compare your risks to those of the heroes in Iraq and Afghanistan, to those of undercover operators in all the risky regions of the world?

The army doesn't get £500.00 per week, either – certainly not for a newly-recruited sprog of twenty, who has the temerity to demand a whole new house as soon as he has joined up – in common with the nursing profession, who think they are entitled to a mansion as soon as look at you. These things have to be earned, by years of hard work and apprenticeship; the culture of 'something for nothing' has taken over the youth of today; they want what they regard as their 'rights' instantly, without any commitment. You are not entitled to anything; the country owes you nothing.

If you complain that you're not 'getting enough', then apply for another job – <u>if</u> you're worth it – and no-one is asking you to be a bloody policeman, anyway. You have an overpaid, steady and secure job, with a thumping good pension at the end of it – unlike the private sector, where nothing is secure, and you are damned lucky to get a pension at all, let alone a good one – and the police retire at an inordinately early age.

The question is, why do these recalcitrant strikes arise? – out of greed; greed and a reckless determination to cause trouble for the government at all costs – an irrational syndrome which raises its ugly head every few years or so throughout the public sector, whether it is teachers, nurses, or even firemen. What, indeed, is this irrational impulse, this desire for self-destruction, even if it means bringing down the establishment with you? Like lemmings you hasten to the scaffold. Obviously the government has to limit pay rises – for a short term; if inflation gets out of hand, there won't be any pay rises at all; an elementary fact, but you insist on shooting yourselves in the foot. Greed, of course, is one motive; envy is another – envy of other professions; as I said, if you don't like being a policeman, get out. Why did you join the police force in the first place? – Because you were too unintelligent to do anything else? – Because it's an easy job? If you like a job, you have to accept its pay structure – it goes <u>with</u> the job; you knew the facts when you started. So why try to commit suicide?

It seems that humanity, when it isn't subverted by greed, <u>has a death-wish</u>. When everything is jogging along Alright, and everyone seems peaceable – then is the moment to pounce; troublemakers will to the fore. Fomenting and stirring the shit is their stock-in trade; whether they actually feel a grievance or not, they deliberately incite unrest among the innocent – and not so innocent; uniformed louts, of whom there are many, are easily persuaded, and the malice of the instigators gives way to the envy and avarice of the instigated. But not content with their own predations, these louts proceed to bully and cajole their more pliant comrades into joining them – sometimes with more subtle methods, such as our old friend, mutual blackmail. These well-versed practitioners weigh in with the subliminal threat that anyone who goes against the grain will have his balls crushed – not a very nice thing, and it works a treat. Poor innocents, who would otherwise not venture a dissenting word, are prevailed upon to espouse the common cause.

Mutual-blackmail is the way society holds itself together, whether collective society or individual societies, such as the police force; everyone intimates to everyone else that 'if you do not toe the line, I will withdraw your "membership"' or, alternatively, 'I'll have the balls off you'. The efficacy of this self-implosive conspiracy can not be doubted.

Where is the element of egotism in all this? It is not hard to find. In these marching, mouthing yobs we have the essence of the opportunistic, ranting bully, out to get as much as he can lay his hands on and to soak the government for every possible, dishonourable penny. All of which he thinks is justified by his own, self-exaggerated worth; what makes him think that an ex-butcher's boy or an erstwhile navvy is entitled to the same salary as a cabinet minister? – which is logically what he is saying, or intimating: 'I am as good as anyone', quite forgetting his origins and the fact that a cabinet minister has earned his pay through years of hard work and dedication – not to mention his natural intelligence and cultural polish. The factor of high responsibility also enters here; what is the average policeman responsible for – apart from farting in the canteen?

The upper echelons in the police service are of course entitled to a higher wage than that of their fat underlings, but they have been persuaded to go along with the march by their own pusillanimous fear of going against the tide of their colleagues' demands – despite their personal reservations. How would it look if the Chief Inspector failed to support his men? He would be <u>extremely</u> unpopular…

The distressing fact of inadequacy in the average human being is perfectly exemplified by the machinations of the militant louts on the one hand and the weak-kneed capitulation of the higher officials on the other; both are in need of a strong dose of educative arse- kicking.

The Indian Tit Wobbler

I had a dream in which there was a circus act, in England – though put on by a lady of a certain Asian origin – where this person appeared to demonstrate the miraculous healing powers of the female Tit. I did not think this was funny, but regarded it with the utmost seriousness; in fact I fell in love with the woman. Within this Tit revolved the world.

I was put out by the apparent Indian origin of this feat – for some reason I wanted desperately for it to be a Western-English – phenomenon – but it proved to have originated from some Asian philosophy.

Perhaps I myself originated from India. And, in the dream, I think the Tit itself was largely a 'red-herring'.

One of the most interesting developments was the appearance of Christ himself, preaching to an English audience; he was demonstrating at the end – though not explicitly – how the powers he exhibited were not of a physical origin but came from some other source – unspecified, but indicated as something mental, if not psychological.

Therefore, the dream was not a flop. This is the first dream in which I have been identified with Christ. Dreams always tell the truth, and invariably involve oneself (although they may also involve other people, these people would be intimately connected with the dreamer – for instance one's family). This is the basic fact about dreams, and also the reason why the thousands of books on this subject – written by posturing psychiatrists – are absolutely useless; they purport to interpret dreams on the basis of archetypal symbols, but because it is impossible to understand this material without having an intimate knowledge of the individual's history, these attempts are doomed to failure. There are indeed universal symbols from which it is possible to interpret the material involved, but these are comparatively uncommon; in any case, even in such an eventuality, it would still be necessary to know the <u>individual angle</u> from which the dream is to be decoded.

I think it was probably Freud who first exposed the inner workings of dreams, along with unconsciousness in general, but in the admittedly limited number of books I have read about the East, the Orientals exhibit a marked lack of awareness of the dream-world – and, indeed, <u>of the unconscious itself</u>. I find it hard to believe that Asian pundits are totally ignorant of these things – after all, their philosophy is <u>based on what emerges from the unconscious</u> – nevertheless, they do not seem to <u>focus</u> on it – <u>and most of their dreams seem to occur in waking life</u>; that is, in their transcendental 'stream of consciousness'. Their 'dream' symbols consist of distinctly conscious ideas; what does this say? In the West we concentrate on the unconscious itself; in the East they apparently concentrate on what is <u>produced</u> by the unconscious. What is the significance? It lies in the dichotomy between experience (unconsciousness) and thought (consciousness); preoccupied by experience as we are in Europe, we turn our attention to two things: practical matters and instinct – in a word, Sensation. Instinct, the basis of experience, relies on the <u>overall function of Sensation</u>; in the developed, or civilized, psyche, sensation is relegated to one of the four more or less differentiated psychological functions; they being thought, emotion, intuition, and, of course, sensation itself. Intuition and emotion are intimately bound up with instinct – or <u>unconscious</u> sensation. The 'overall function' of Sensation is essentially unconscious, but the <u>conscious, or abstract</u>, sensation is a tool specifically designed for the pursuit of art: a combination of instinct and thought (or abstraction).

Practical matters also demand a combination of instinct and thought – ideally – but <u>practical actions</u>, as opposed to <u>directed, or abstract</u>, actions are characterized by sensation. In science, the quintessential area of practicality, both sensation and thought are present, but unlike art, science does not possess instinct or intuition, and certainly not emotion, all of which art possess in abundance; science is a one-horse function. The artist is inspired by all the unconscious functions, which, as we have seen, add up to Sensation, plus the thinking function; but it is a fact, unacknowledged by Jung, who actually invented the term 'abstract sensation', <u>that thinking is not necessarily conscious</u> – since even animals can think (although science uses instinct, it is not a significant factor in that discipline).

The Asian preoccupation is, of course, with consciousness, or thought – whether directed or otherwise – their thought being, in fact extremely conscious; that is, in the case of <u>Eastern pundits</u>. who are the only significant element in their society, the rest being, for the most part, ignorant peasants. One might think, in con- comitance with this, that the East lacks individuality – which it does, the intelligentsia being confined to a few members of that body. The Asians, most of them – at least, those maintaining the official position – would not recognize individuality as a valid conception, their orientation being towards unity, not plurality, which is a Western idea. Whether or not there are a few enlightened thinkers who espouse the idea of individuality, I do not know, but it is quite possible; nevertheless, the Eastern psyche is inimicably opposed to any such orientation – and it is the psyche we are concerned with.

The Eastern philosophy is directed towards introversion (again, a Jungian term) which I associate essentially with consciousness, the extroverted position being, itself, directed towards instinct or sensation, which is basically unconscious. While extroversion can obviously include thought, is that thought actually possessed of true consciousness? In so far as thought is 'directed' – that is, informed – it is of course in the conscious mode, but in the objective, or extroverted, function thinking is bent towards the task at hand, and though it is instructed by the mind, this brand of awareness is not conscious; as in animals, thinking is not necessarily contained in such a medium.

This is the reason why the East is orientated to consciousness, while excluding the subliminal.

Sex

The idea that sex is for pleasure is a total, and disastrous, illusion.

THE THIRD ELEMENT

The Anglo-Saxon word 'fuck' was originally invented to convey two meanings: one, the process of giving or receiving pleasure, and, two, the expression of spiritual regard, both given and received.

It may not be immediately obvious that spirituality is conveyed in a word that has become synonymous with crudity, but originally- and this has been whispered in my ear – the Anglo-Saxons intended the word to convey the two meanings simultaneously; i.e. as Love'. Now, love does indeed consist of both pleasure and spirit; it does not consist of 'sex', which means, specifically, pleasure – usually illicit pleasure – and specifically not spirit. Psychiatrists have been telling us, ever since the end of the nineteenth century, that spirit is a bad thing, because it spoils pleasure And because psychiatrists are schizophrenics, they are unaware of the dichotomy in their own mentalities; to wit, that if one is asked to make love, or fuck, one needs to employ both spirit and pleasure, because it is impossible to fuck anyone without giving and receiving at the same time: one's cunt and one's cock (two other Anglo-Saxon words) would either not <u>receive</u> any pleasure or not <u>give</u> it, thus rendering the situation into a fiasco, or defeating its original purpose – which is, of course, as Sigmund Freud has tried so hard to convince us, to produce a dirty good shag. Now, a dirty good shag depends specifically on the absence of spirit; pleasure it certainly has, but – and this is where schizophrenia comes in – when both partners are receiving pleasure under such circumstances, it is impossible to determine whether either of them is actually giving it; in point of fact, <u>neither</u> of them is giving it, and it is only received by virtue of auto-erotic self suggestion – in other words, by illusion;

the illusion that one is receiving attention from one's nefarious partner. Apart from the somewhat limited contact between cock and cunt, the two 'partners' are totally divorced, their minds operating in fantasy; and, imprisoned in their own fantastic world, they are unaware of who is shagging whom or whether anyone is actually being shagged anyway. In this twilight world of schizophrenia, therefore, anything goes – and it only comes by dint of much hard pushing and shoving in the locality of the genitals. The result might be considered satisfying, however, if all you are after is a frenetic and dirtily achieved orgasm.

But of course, Dr Psycho maintains that sex was invented for the sole purpose of attaining an orgasm, essentially restricted to the genitals, genital-sex knowing no experience, or sensation, in the rest of the body; satisfaction is not felt beyond that frenzied area. So, neither in body nor mind, does illicit sex exist – except, where mind is concerned, in obscene and destructive fantasies which have literally nothing to do with genuine sexuality.

All this can be attributed to the influence of Sigmund Freud – the Father of Sex, but not of love. Although he recognized the importance of love in the psyche as a whole, the existence of love as the purpose and controlling factor of sexuality entirely escaped him. He dissociated sex from love and presented it as a function independent of those of the rest of the psyche, a conviction supported by G.I. Gurdjieff who, unfortunately for the followers he misled, was governed by his own psychological function of sensation, which in some mentalities does involve the isolation of the 'sex-function' – including its isolation from love.

Now, God informed me before I came down to earth, <u>that spirit is the purpose of sex and that pleasure is the means</u>. It would seem, therefore, that where man is going wrong is in getting things arse- ways about, under the instructions of psychiatry and those who call themselves 'intellectuals'. Of course, man listens to these authorities open-mouthed, not having a mind of his own, though, truth to tell, his mentors haven't any sort of a mind at all. So, then, the blind leading the blind, we are precipitated into a state of mental anarchy whose distinguishing feature is universal Masturbation. Masturbating day and night, on the job or off it, women as well as men, <u>we live</u>

<u>in a world of total fantasy</u>. Grandmothers and Grandfathers, as long as they can get their leg over, fall into the same category: contained totally within their infantile fantasies, they claw at each other, in their attempts at sexual intercourse, succeeding only in remaining faithful to their adolescent immaturity. Reality they see not – a bum here, a tit there, and a what's-it over there, totally uncombined, totally unintegrated: this is not a body – it is certainly not a mind – it is simply a pre-pubertal glimpse of the chaos within a child's mind – unformed sexuality, pervading society like a rampant disease. This is the civilization wrought upon us by modernism.

Make no mistake about it, love is essential to sex, and not optional, as Dr Psycho pontificates. Thanks to the Dr's ego-driven, and schizophrenically expressed beliefs, twenty-first century man and woman are perpetually tortured by the schism between lust and love; though this is the age-old problem, it has been exacerbated out of all proportion by psychiatry's unwonted interference. The ignorance of this body, foisted on us by pure conceit, has led us to abandon our birthright of self-respect – specifically recommended on the assumption that sex is intended to be dirty – that we should enjoy it; and the dirtier it is, the more we should enjoy it. Of course, if man could think for himself he would know this is not true, but persuaded by the authority of newspapers and television, who have rallied to Dr Psycho's cause, he lives in the constant conviction that the more he lowers his trousers, the more he is going to enjoy himself – regardless, of course, of is wife's reservations (this, also, being one of the doctor's recommendations). The belief that 'sex is for fun', which flies in the face of God's commands, and also in the face of man's own sense of shame, has prompted society to dedicate itself to the pursuit of evil; where there is no need for restraint, we do not restrain ourselves, and because the overriding purpose of sex is apparently 'to enjoy ourselves', the restraining influence of spirit is not allowed to interfere. And love, the original inspiration and goal of sex – that is, according to God – expires unwanted.

This we see every day, all around us, in the tight-trousered bums and flaunted tits proffered for the express purpose of drawing the dirtiest possible shag. And all because Dr Psycho has told us to do it. The contagion spreads, like flies around shit, from schoolroom to dance-hall, inspiring the dropping of pants in all directions, in the determination to get that all-consuming orgasm – a seizure of the fanny so pleasurable, apparently, that all sense of decency is frenziedly rejected – Just what the doctor ordered, and in sweaty, frenetic couplings across the land, male and female shag their way into the devil's own Piss-Kitchen.

And they like it because it <u>is</u> evil. Innocent pleasure has become evil because of the withdrawal of its tending partner, <u>and it has developed into the mad desire to destroy even God and Creation itself: rend down those curtains surrounding the Hole of Holies!</u>

'Just like shitting', as the man said, and this excretory function has been confused with sex, in the mind of man, ever since Sigmund Freud defecated on the idea of natural instinct – which was designed to lead us, mistakenly it seems, to consult our sexual consciences.

<u>Sex is not to be enjoyed.</u>

Pleasure is, of course, love, and love pleasure, as Fanny Hill said; but, as she also added, 'love is the only thing that ennobles it'. This paradoxical statement is actually very profound – though the lady herself was actually entirely unconscious of that – in that the whole relationship of opposites is essentially one of paradox. Take on board the fact that life itself is Paradox. And from that will ensue our understanding of the meaning of sex.

Right in the heart of pleasure, we find spirit; right in the heart of spirit, we find pleasure; and right in the heart of both of them, we find Love – Love, the king-pin. But think not that the element of spirit is any greater than that of pleasure; <u>pleasure is. indeed, the purpose of love;</u> the end to which it is directed and the means by which we achieve it; <u>while spirit is also the purpose of love</u>, it is specifically the means by which we are guided through it; without spirit we would be rudderless in the ocean of lust.

Lust, indeed, is actually love – love gone wrong, through the withdrawal of spirit. But it is nevertheless innocent in its origins, being in fact the very inspiration to love: without it, we simply would not want to make love. So, without the desire to shag you, I would not shag you; and you would not have the satisfaction of being shagged.

And shag you, is what I intend to do.

THE IDEAL STATE, AND PURPOSE. OF LOVE…

A Letter Addressed To Venus, My Muse:

In the determination to love me, she undresses, slowly and deliberately before me, and presents herself, completely naked, for my inspection. Running my eye over her inviting young body, I gulp nervously in contemplation of what I am going to do with her; shall I fuck her straight away, without much circumspection – which she would welcome, as she is now pretty urgent – or shall I prolong her crisis to induce even further pleasure? While I am hesitantly debating my procedure, however, Venus herself decides the matter for me. Lying on her back and signalling her intentions with the most amorous entreaty of her so-beautiful eyes, she parts her lovely thighs, opening herself to me like a flower yearning for the kiss of the sun. And being the gentleman I am, I approach her with all the ardour she has aroused, and enter her, then and there, to prove it. Prone and yielding, the woman I love gives herself up to me, her master, in our mutual rapture.

Thus the abandoned Whore, consecrated by the overwhelming love of the Mother; the one, pleasure itself, the other, pure spirit. Little all the while, little in love – that is how we love each other: 'Except ye be as little children, ye shall not enter the kingdom of heaven'. And the kingdom of heaven awaits us, not just in our littleness, but also in the magnificence conferred on us by our modesty.

For pleasure is the name of the game, or so I would hope. Most dirty buggers, however, would assume that pleasure is actually the purpose, proceeding on that basis to fuck the living daylights out of her without even an introduction. Now, I myself, being a decent sort of chap, would no doubt fuck the living daylights out of her likewise, but I would generally not omit to introduce myself; for politeness is politeness, and the etiquette of sex has it that you are not allowed to fuck a woman unless you very definitely love her. Pleasure may be pleasure, and thank God for that, but it cannot displace spirit, and most certainly cannot supersede our reason for fucking, which is simply the requirement to barnstorm our beloved into the delirium of Absolute Love – from which there is no return, for, once having been there, Milady has no intention of returning to a mundane world; we hope, therefore that, ideally, her swain will never let her go, but ply her with perfect devotion for the rest of her days – if possible with no relapse into normality.

This is God's design for man. In a constant state of high tumescence, then, the happy couple are expected to remain within love indefinitely; the world may continue around them on its giddy course, but these two have united in a place of Knowledge, issuing from themselves, which will sustain them forever in blissful disregard of earthly cares. Knowledge knows all, and consequently resolves all – which is, on consideration, our ultimate desire.

The passion of pleasure: love given, love received.

There is no hint of dissociation, or exaggeration, in our pleasure. We are Us, and we are Love; that is all. Pleasure, love, and passion: All in One.

And passion is why I fuck you – that word, passion, uniting pleasure with love, and lifting it right out of pleasure into love, thus extinguishing it. <u>Pleasure must die, so that the spiritual body may live.</u> And, so transformed, pleasure will yet remain pleasure, but offered to God, and living in god's realm where there is, after all, <u>no pleasure</u>: the Incomprehensible Paradox right at the heart of being.

This knowledge will save all from the ravages of pleasure. Everyone does in fact urgently want to learn about it – even whores sold to lust. Salvation awaits us all, <u>because we all want it.</u>

———————

In that word, 'fuck', I am uniting pleasure with spirit; first of all dissociating them by withdrawing the unity of Love, which they had initially, and now, after aeos of travail, in which the word 'fuck' became very disreputable, I have established the basis of their future reconciliation – within, again, Love. Love was – Love is. Unity, being disintegrated, now becomes re-integrated in Union, conscious love ensuing.

Seventy-five per cent of the people in Western Europe are guilty of sexual perversion – a conservative estimate. I do not mean homosexuality or lesbianism, <u>but the simple fact of downright dirty behaviour.</u> Whether this is by will or whether involuntary, I do not quite know, but certainly it is wanton and wilful.

Sexual perversion, in this sense of the word, is invariably caused by <u>dissociation or exaggeration</u>. When I observe a girl, I don't look at her bum or her tits directly; this would be to dissociate them from the rest of the body, and to exaggerate them at the same time. It is a disgusting, but unfortunately true, fact that most men see only the bums or the tits – <u>without</u> the rest of the body; the vast majority of men see a woman as, simply, a bum, a pair of tits, and the crumpet as the focal point: truly a 'sexual object', or objects. How many times have I witnessed this – and it goes without saying that the more a woman omits to wash herself, the better…

Thus the sewer within man's mind in the twenty-first century, to which woman is unwillingly, or willingly, subjected. The focal point of a woman's body is, or should be, the eyes; they are the window of the soul, where the woman lives. Her face, also, reflects her being – not just her other appurtenances, such as the bosom, which is the direct expression of her love, not just her personal being; the more fulsome a woman's breasts, the more you may be sure of the warmth, or generosity, of her love. Treat her, therefore, with respect. Her bosom is her love, and, its beauty, her loveliness.

Looked at as a whole, woman's body retains its natural integrity, so furnishing her with the dignity which both she and her body deserve. So, gracefully and elegantly, she conducts herself through congress, undressed only to be dressed again in the finer robes of sacred nakedness.

Parsifal's Proposition to Venus

My Beloved;

After taking your knickers off, in the most deliberate manner possible, I will proceed to fuck you. Don't be offended, because this Anglo-Saxon word was designed to express love – and it is very effective, especially in conveying what I have in mind for you; which is precisely this: lying you on your back, where you will become shamelessly abandoned to my love – indeed to Love itself – I will force an entry and submit you to a glorious and very satisfying fucking. God put woman on earth to be submissive, but this submission must be prefaced by resistance; though woman wishes all the while to be overcome, man can only exert himself against her <u>if she first resists</u>. Thus the roles of man and woman are defined, and despite the beliefs of 'womens' lib' the man is for dominance and the woman is for submission; man leads, woman follows. This has been the inalienable law since history began, and will not be changed by Emily Pankhurst's recalcitrant antics; no person ever did greater harm to the cause of women. If this law did not hold, why would I be fucking you now?

So, on your back – the essential position for all women – you invite me to have my wicked way with you – and by God it is wicked; my designs for you would certainly not be countenanced by the Pope.

Holding you tightly within my arms, so that no harm will ever come to you, I propose to render you into a quivering bundle of joy:

<u>Myself</u>, pushing and shoving within you, and drawing your little heart into mine:

'Come ever nearer to me, my darling, and I will show you the ecstasies of heaven! For, in that little place of yours rests the universe, and God sends to you, there, the knowledge of all.'

<u>You</u>, in ecstasy:

'Fuck me, fuck me! Give me all the arduous devotion of which you are so capable; and never stop! (if you do, I shall be most frustrated)'.

<u>Myself:</u> 'Closer, closer! Let me stir your innards to the utmost crescendo of life!'

<u>You,</u> in an extreme of urgency:

'Oh, oh! Fuck the living daylights out of me!'

So, your passion – as released by me. Caressing you above, and delighting you below, this is how I proceed, bringing heart and body together- I, the Reconciler of all Opposites.

And by combining the needs of both spirit and pleasure we come, ourselves, finally together, breathless after all that hectic effort, yet sublime in our knowledge of each other. In that one, final moment, we witnessed Eternity; we knew the presence of God – adding, greatness to our little cause.

But, always proceeding through Love: first, last, and foremost. You can't get a girl's knickers down without approaching her from spirit, first – <u>in</u> the act, and <u>as a result of</u> the act.

The passion implied in the word 'fuck', which I chose deliberately, is mid-way between spirit and pleasure, being synonymous with love but carrying a slightly different meaning. Passion is the active expression of love, and the act of love determines just that: love. Love being above all else, spirit and pleasure, being mere opposites, fade into insignificance. So, the mysterious Third Element, rising between, and above, all its constituent parts – and enveloping them in its all-containing beauty.

You and I know nothing, finally, but the all-consuming passion of Love itself. And so your knickers drop away to reveal only that one thing: the place of Love, and Love alone.

'You and I will fuck forever', you confide in me. – So saying, you lie down on the floor and lift your skirt up, displaying your undying love for me to the world, in your resplendent parts.

We are Love, and Love only. When we are in a high state of pleasure, we are never away from Love; Love is with us, within us, and all around us.

There is so much perverted sex about – that is, dissociated and exaggerated – <u>that no-one is aware of it</u>; if you are all in the same boat, the fact that everybody stinks isn't apparent. And this submersion in unconsciousness is deliberate; no-one is prepared to condemn anyone else – a mutually perpetuating confidence-trick whereby, 'If you do not give me away, I will not give you away'. And anyone who breaks this universal law is 'sent to

Coventry' for betraying his fellows, which I have personally experienced. Sunk within this inescapable morass, the truth never emerges.

Although people are undoubtedly going to be rabidly aroused against me, I do not anticipate a corporate legal challenge – a few million pigs aren't likely to sue anyone.

The causes of this pathological behaviour are unknown and unreported, and I am here to make them known and to report them.

Unmarried whores, married whores – all are prepared to take their pants off for the purpose of experiencing a dirty bit of fun – as directed by psychology, whether consciously or otherwise; the evil genius of Freud presides over it from beyond the grave – all the more evil for being unwitting. Being faced with the preliminary fact of psychological intervention, all men and women have become convinced, despite their instinctive doubts, that sex is here to stay and had better be enjoyed; that is its evident purpose, and woe betide anyone who goes against the popular trend. No-one, apparently, has the guts to stand up and resist it, preferring to sacrifice his own self-respect on two counts: first, that he is a coward, and second that he is determined to roll in the shit – for the sake of it. The one God-given fact of all – the isolated gift of self- respect – has been surrendered in the face of physical attack and the desire to commit pure evil – against oneself. Self-respect was set up to combat all attempts to assail the integrity of the Self, in the name of truth, honesty, and the sanctity of life itself; this sanctity is, above all, what is being assaulted. God will not forgive you for that.

So we have lorry drivers selecting their molls for a dirty good screw behind the dustbins, cock-eyed trollops inviting the nearest letcher to rattle their only-too receptive fannies into a dizzy delight, and, in every doorway, mid the complicit shadows, the attempt of the female sex to induce a frantic orgasm by sucking, to the best of their ability, every ounce of sperm from a drunkard's cock.

And yet we have the Archbishop of Canterbury telling us that these women – 'working girls', I believe is the term – are actually angels in distress, not responsible for what they are doing –

though they can see a man's chopper Alright – and that they have become prostitutes for the sole purpose of making money – pleasure, we assume, having nothing to do with it. Far from being forced into their plight – by economic necessity! – these hellions remove their sweaty underwear, all day and all night, purely because they are nymphomaniacs! – Every man's dream, of course – and the sweatier and smellier, the better. The fond illusions of society's do-gooders do not alter the horrific reality of illicit sex – which is not just illicit but actually has nothing to do with sex at all – the very concept is laughable – being the desperate expression of a sickness affecting the whole of civilization. Whores are whores because they feel whoredom where it is felt.

This is the wrath of God, speaking.

Upper-class tarts, like Trinny and Fanny, are usually the worst, somehow having persuaded the B.B.C. to employ them as 'sex experts' – this term, apparently, conferring social acceptability on what I would have thought was a most unholy calling. Of course, as we know, amateur whores are even more accomplished than their professional sisters. These two representatives of the ruling elite give us the benefit of their extensive experience in demonstrations of how women should dress and behave in order to entrap the opposite sex. 'Stick your bum out as far as possible; walk down the street with the maximum salaciousness – that's right, sway your hips, as if you are trying to catch a fish – and make sure your tits are in full prominence'. All this with the egotistical confidence that they have been chosen to perform an essential service! Their only service is in persuading otherwise innocent women that love is not relevant in sexual affairs which require only a devotion to an immediate orgasm. And so, orgasmically primed, these unfortunates make their way to their husbands in order to demand attention to their very urgent needs; how they behave on the bus, I don't know.

Trinny and Fanny, of course, will no doubt consult their solicitors with a view to suing me. Unfortunately, I have no money.

ORGASM

That little, short-lived moment. Short-lived, did you say? That 'little moment' contains <u>every</u> moment – it lasts for Eternity; all moments in one moment, <u>all time</u> in one moment; realized in the Eternal Present. And we would know – or see – this <u>if we were conscious</u>. So let us become conscious.

One way to do it is to hold back this very, ultimate moment as long as possible – until it hurts; do without it, if you can. Suffering produces consciousness, something which is, or should be, known in the catholic church; for celibacy is designed for this purpose; along with its sister goal of Love, Consciousness was the express aim of Popery.

All archbishops, canons, and canonicals will be trained in this venture; for, owing to human susceptibility – as we have seen – priests must learn to master a woman before taking the vow, otherwise they will go wanking and buggaring into the night.

Without the consciousness provided by suffering, how are priests to produce the compassion needed for their 'flock'? How are these potential Parsifals to know, or feel, anything? One moment becomes All moments only through the intervention of divine enlightenment.

As the obverse of the world that God holds in his hand, let that little drop of spunk, emitted by your orgasm, contain everything.

<u>THE CURE</u>

<u>Now to the main purpose of this essay. As you should all know, but don't, I have not come to this earth for nothing; it is my specific duty to clear this farrago of cock-titillators and fanny-rattlers off the face of the earth. God's house will not be used by usurers.</u>

THE SPIRITUAL-BODY

The Twenty First Century declaration for the evolution of the sexual phenomenon consists of the introduction of the 'Spiritual Body' into man's psyche. This latest dispensation from God will change human sexual behaviour forever – in particular, relieving man of his very nasty erotic habits. Perhaps the most significant thing of all is that the necessity of the act of intercourse itself will be obviated; while the substituted Spiritual Body does not – <u>or need not</u> – involve the sexual act as we know it, it leaves the door open to the sexual experience without the contact of the genitals – though if desirable, this could be included. All options are open.

Pleasure is certainly felt, with or without genital contact; no-one is losing out. The watchword is 'Sublimation'. Man's all-compelling enslavement to the physical side of life – to the very existence of flesh – is over at one stroke. From now on we are psychological beings.

The psyche – or mind – contains both the body and the mentality; it is a mistake to equate the mentality with the mind, of which it is only a part.

Annie is a very passionate girl. In her we see, on the one hand, her physical passion, on the other, her spiritual passion: the flesh, and the spirit. This most attractive young woman, though not conventionally beautiful, exhibits, more than most, the very unconventional beauty of Emotion; that is to say, her face displays the evidence of a commitment to Passion – the halfway-house between the normal concerns of spirit and flesh. Passion comes from the heart, the location of the true sexual experience, poised mid-way between the genitals and the head, the genitals being ultra-flesh, and the head being ultra-spirit.

Emotion, or Passion, passing through the body – the <u>vessel</u> of Emotion – takes up, from one end, spirit and from the other, flesh, <u>combining them, within itself, as the Third Element</u>. This Third Element is the essence of the 'Spiritual Body'.

THE THIRD ELEMENT. THROUGH THE ULTIMATE EXPERIENCE

A little old lady, the other day, stoned out of her mind, offered me the chance to have my chopper cut off free of charge. Now, I know I could get this done on the National Health, but quite frankly, I would prefer her attentions, and of course, the most salubrious scenario would be the receipt of this operation from your own lover, particularly when she is a voluptuous young blonde. In the heat of that very singular moment – your very private parts being severed by your best, and most devoted, friend

– indeed, in the most attentively erotic manner possible – surely you would experience the ultimate pleasure? What more could you want from that sacrifice of all sacrifices?

One thing you could want is the metaphysical knowledge of what you were doing. On the one hand we have destruction – the operation – on the other hand we have creation – the orgasm; between the two we have the Schism, assuming there is an unbridgeable gap. If the unbridgeable Schism is to vanish, it must be transformed into a relationship, in other words, into two complementaries, opposites being complementary in an ideal state of relationship. The relationship itself is the Third Element – <u>including even the Schism.</u>

But the raw material of all this – the opposites themselves – is the contrast between destruction and creation – two very irreconcilable qualities – yet not so irreconcilable: is not destruction but one remove from creation? – <u>Are they not identical?</u> Just as Life and Death fuse into one, under similar circumstances, so destruction – Death – and creation – Life, are finally brought together: the Phoenix of creation rises eternally from the Pyre of destruction, and, ultimately, they know each other in one Pyrotechnical Moment.

<u>Think not that you will get away with identifying spirit with pleasure, or pleasure with spirit: the whole of evolution forbids it. I, in my Second Coming, know all too well the Schism of all things Natural – become, most almightily, unnatural: Natural Man is dead, only to be resurrected in the Union of Opposites – no longer the Unity of former times.</u>

<u>So, take on board the requirements of evolution, and of your own psyche. To be, or not to be: that is the thinking question.</u>

Always approach a woman, first, with Love, in which all things are united. But when you shag, you shag with spirit and pleasure first of all separately, then you bring them together – in one, indistinguishable Moment, where pleasure exists separately, but <u>does not exist.</u>

So, the Imponderable Paradox of our human – or divine – nature.

<u>There is no going back to Unity; that is now denied us, forbidden us; which is why Buddhism is in such a parlous state –</u>

indeed, a time- warp. Christianity holds the way forward, into the future – Union – born of a desirable, though necessarily disastrous, Duality – a real Duality. Dualism may have its drawbacks, as has plurality, but they both exist, and have a right and purpose in existing. The fact that plurality is inconvenient for Buddhist thought does not mean it is an illusion – unless you consider that the whole of the exterior world is an illusion (which I can prove is not the case). Where Buddhists go wrong is in equating the exterior world with the physical world – an understandable problem in the light of their centrifugal psyche.

In place of 'Christian', I would put forward the name 'Antonian' – meaning the 'Antonian' religion, as I do not espouse, beyond a certain extent, the Christian religion itself; the Antonian is built upon the relics of the Christian religion, with smatterings of every other religion thrown in as well. This should mollify any residual egotism lurking around the world.

[Without spirit, we would have not the pleasure; without pleasure, we would have not the spirit].

[We do not desire each others' bodies; we desire each other].

Returning to the 'Spiritual-Body':

Much as I regret my debarment from the indulgence of physical desire, this can all be sublimated in the emotional state: a compromise between, and a combination of, spirit and body – resolved in the Heart. The heart is where Christ proposes to conduct his programme for the world – essentially through imagination; a process which at the moment only Christ can produce. Imagination, as Christ is putting it forward, is a vastly different thing to the so-called 'imagination' present in the conventional idea. I have come here to revolutionize all conventions and concepts, imagination being one of them. Imagination, therefore, is a free-ranging ability to 'see all'; imagination sees everything. ('Free-ranging' is a very adequate, Jungian phrase). This is what the faculty always has consisted of, but has remained unrecognized until now. It also contains reason, contrary to all accepted belief.

Imaginative thinking is the way forward for the modern world – perhaps Christ's most valuable gift. In it is resolved the whole question of the inner and outer lives, these being brought together in the Spiritual-Body: a combination of subjective and objective factors, <u>which relieves one of the necessity of living and working within the physical body,</u> unless one chooses to do so – in other words, among other things, one is able to make love conducted on an emotional though not physical, basis, <u>mid-way between body and spirit: including both, but, essentially, not of both.</u>

[See 'Sublimation', from the preface to 'The Knowledge Of Everything'; also 'Transubstantiation' from the essay, 'Sudanese Blasphemy Crisis' ('Knowledge Of Everything') also 'Secret Of Desire', again from 'Knowledge Of Everything'.]

An Amorous Frolic

The creasing of the upper thigh,
Under the welt of a black stocking
The swelling, strategic areas
Beneath a nice, black negligee -
The endearing and fervent scent
Of a woman in her amorous embrace:
These things, so intimate,
Are not to be forgotten.

Abandoning the negligee,
She clasps her hands behind her head,
Offering her full-bosomed self to my regard,
And, shifting her hips – not her backside -
Slightly, she disposes herself
In a more inviting position;
What more could a man stand!
Such response this brings,
That I am moved to a sturdy vigour
In those regions below the belt;
And what more could a ladies' champion do
Than 'take advantage' of a very critical situation!
Inspired to an ardent clinch, therefore,
We enjoy the ecstatic mode
Of Love's transporting ways

[Masturbation pervades all aspects of life.]

[Woman is born whole, and so she doesn't need to travel through the journey of masturbation to become mature].

Teenage boys must 'masturbate' (to use a nasty term) for a long time before they can achieve sexual maturity. 'Making love to your hand', therefore, is a necessary and indispensable preliminary to making love to your later sweetheart – who will not despise you for it – especially when it produces such beautiful experiences for herself!

So let us go wanking.

A Note On The Cosmic Physiology Of Sexuality

You and I experience the knowledge of each other in that conveyancing medium called 'pleasure'. Pleasure is designed for the express purpose of enabling us to know each other in and through love. In itself, pleasure does not exist, on the basis that it represents, quintessentially, the illusion of the physical world, being used for the purpose of love, and that is all; the physical world is set up to facilitate intercourse between the opposites, after which it retires, redundant, and vanishes into the ether from which it came.

Nevertheless, I can only know you, I can only give you love, through that febrile tissue of pleasure; so it is extremely useful, but as all functions, it has no other reality except as the function it actually is, limited to itself and shortly to be deprived of its existence when viewed through the all-seeing eye of consciousness – the product of love.

Let us honour pleasure, therefore, but let us not make it a god.

Desire being passion, we find ourselves committed to pleasure: why else would you desire to be fucked? (the word, fuck, being much more beautiful than the derogatory term of shag). Being so passionate in your experience of pleasure (why else would I love you?) you force me to acknowledge the very sanguine fact that pleasure, far from being restricted to the genitals, extends over the whole body and particularly into the mind – where it comes from. Being felt, perhaps, most intensely in the genitals, the sheer joy, the passion of pleasure, originates within the mind, <u>and proceeds from it</u>, reverberating around your rapturous body, and, only as a last resort, penetrating to the genitals; the focal point, however, is not in this transient area but in the eyes. The eyes reflect the music of the soul, or mind: <u>the pleasure centre</u>; from where it proceeds again around the body and returns to the mind, and back eternally, on its constant round, increasing in intensity as it goes. This climactic journey is facilitated, at each of its stations, by the transforming spirit of libido, which effects the necessary paradox, turning spirit into pleasure and back again. Without this constant transformation, the opposites would become fixated in their own exaggerated and isolated position – hence resulting in the pathological paralysis which we know as 'perversion' – a condition which affects most people in Western civilization and which perpetuates, by its paralyzing influence, its fatal, fantastic illusion, reducing even intercourse to the permanent immaturity of masturbation. Masturbation remains in most of us until death.

Where is this Centre, the Soul? Is it in the head? Is it in the heart? Is it in the body? Or is it in the genitals? It is in all these places, and far beyond them, emanating from the outer reaches of the universe – <u>and at the same time, from the very centre of it</u>. This is the experience of God: the source of all pleasure and passion – combined at once in Love, the true purpose, and sole justification for, <u>a pleasure that, finally, does not even exist</u>, having played a yet noble part in the creation of the greatest climax known to the life of us humans.

So, therefore, do not decry pleasure – nor, if you are a psychiatrist, the opposite, spirit. Taken together these two form not just the basis of love, <u>but the foundation of all knowledge</u>: the knowledge of Good and Evil, the observation of Essence and Existence, forming between them the ultimate consciousness of Metaphysics. This hybrid method of knowing and seeing is the goal of our existence, furnishing us by its very function with the means of finding it: the Paradox which draws us on through the daylight of Masculinity into the mysterious night of the Feminine.

And thus, all men and women come together in the celebration of Eternal Life upon earth.

Only by will can we reverse the deadly influence of masturbation; only by taking upon ourselves the lengthy journey of maturation do we stand any chance of freeing ourselves from its stranglehold. <u>The application of will for this purpose requires prolonged consciousness, that in itself being acquired only by painstaking experience in the very maturation process.</u> Consciousness confers knowledge; knowledge cures.

We have to come to know ourselves, through honesty and the attempt to abandon ego, ego being the very thing which blinds us to reality – even the reality of sex. Without coming to know ourselves, and consequently our sexual nature, sexuality will never develop, and we will be left behind in our masturbatory prison. The one thing, above all, which qualifies maturity, is Love. Without love, woman would not make love to man, nor man to woman; the expression is 'making love', not 'making sex', and the attempt to substitute sex for love lies at the bottom of that monstrous evil called 'modernism', unleashed on us by, among others, Pankhurst and Freud. Freud ended love itself, Pankhurst ended femininity – the very quality needed most in love, by both women and men. Loveless, the twentieth century proceeded with the clarion cry, 'We do not need woman, we do not need God!' Both God and woman died on the cross of modernist untruth; and love died with them.

GERMAINE GREER

This Australian-born example of perverted womanhood has bestridden the stage of modern sexuality for nigh on fifty years (she looks old enough, anyway). Lined and be-wrinkled, yet still thinking herself young enough to invite the whole male sex into bed with her, she holds forth in the media as the champion of sex-without- love. This is her manifesto, declared from the outset in the words… 'When you wake up in bed with *someone*…' This says it all; this is her philosophy: 'Shag all and everything', without a care in the world – why should you have? – you're not committed to anybody. That would defeat the purpose of it, anyway, which appears to be to demonstrate the deliberate extirpation, not just of spirit, but also of any personal connotation whatever.

Without the person to do the shagging, no shag can take place, and in place of the shag we are left with, of course, masturbation. This, in all but name, is what she seeks; the withdrawal of personal involvement leaves the sex act without a focal point – or a purpose; the classic case of adolescent self-abuse.

So we are left with the schizophrenic identity of, on the one hand, an ignoramus masquerading as an intellectual, and on the other, a man masquerading as a woman.

The 'Feminist Movement' having actually removed all traces of femininity from women in general and from the act of love in particular, we are minus the precious influence of the feminine; there is no womanhood, and consequently no love, and no civilization either. For civilization is built on Love and the Feminine Principle. These are the consequences of Emily Pankhurst's exhibitionist tendencies. And, in passing, there has never been a convincing case made out for the right of women to vote. 'Why should men have the exclusive right to vote? This is unfair to women'. For anything to be unfair to women, you have first to prove that women are on an equal footing to men; Nature invented women with the express intention of their being inferior. Men, by design, have always been the leaders, but, in my opinion, this does not make women actually inferior: they would only appear so as the result of Pankhurst's interference, upon which the ugly head of ego reared itself. Previously, Nature had managed to ensure that woman had <u>no</u> ego; that salutary fact had sustained woman throughout evolution, and by God's purpose as well as Nature's, man was very often restrained from going to war on this same account. Woman's lack of ego has enabled her to counsel her opposite sex on matters so grave as aggression and sexuality, and it is the purpose of evolution to create civilization on the very basis of man's adoption of the feminine trait. Thus, if you subtract femininity from civilization, we revert to savagery. And the primitive savage we see today in the person of woman – demanding everything, from the right to work to the right to do away with their unborn child – was created by the declaration that women should assert themselves in the role of men, quite contrary to their nature.

It is an undoubted fact also, that, in contradiction to his natural tendencies, man has succumbed to the very quality that made civilization possible: the feminine trait. So effeminate is Western man at this moment, that our civilization will not survive an attack from the Muslim East, the Muslim religion never having attempted to force femininity on its own people. Whether you consider this to be a good thing or not, it has enabled the Muslims to defeat every Christian effort to overcome them from the Crusades onward. As the Arabs constantly point out to me, on looking at Western culture, the women are all like men, and the men are all like women; which has a distinct advantage, I suppose, in the event of attack, where men will cower in the kitchen while the women go forth sword in hand – and God help those bloody Muslims!

I have come here to teach the British nation to fight, and the first thing I am going to do is to get hold of every vicar and archbishop in the land and set them up in the ring with boxing gloves on. I'll have them fighting like heroes – and I'll throw in a few psychiatrists as well. God never told womankind to don their husbands' trousers; unfortunately, Mrs Thatcher thought he did, and as a result we were treated to the unwelcome spectacle of this redoubtable woman taking on the Russians on behalf of the vacillating British male. If my Father had come out of retirement, he would have married that woman, and he would have proceeded to tame her by taking her pants down and smacking her little bottom. Femininity having thus been restored, the happy couple would have retreated to a bungalow in Blackpool, where we would never have heard from her again – but we'd have lost a good prime minister…

All women need to be beaten, and any impertinent challenge to their husband's authority must be put down. Man rules, woman obeys – the natural law ever since Christ last bestrode the earth. All you modern pansies be warned: a woman does not respect a man if he respects her; the greatest respect a man can show a woman is not to respect her. Woman needs to be taken, not asked – if, that is, she is a natural woman, and hasn't been subverted by Pankhurst's disastrous attentions. I have fucked thousands of women into the experience of heaven – precisely because I forced them. They wanted to be fucked, of course, but they wouldn't submit unless they were sure that their lover intended to dominate them; the very resistance they put up is intended to be overcome.

The roles of men and women have been reversed, and despite the beliefs of the church and Mary Whitehouse, God did not intend this change of gender in his virile world. The Archbishop of Canterbury's skirt hides a meagre pair of testicles.

Women have no business, either, being nuns. Nuns invariably reek of decaying flesh; as they have never been fucked, their bodies have gone rancid, and being therefore unnourished, they stink; God does not welcome a malodorous female in his bed. The 'Brides Of Christ' are rejected.

Men and women are put on earth for only two purposes: to fight and to fuck; but I wouldn't fuck a nun if I was paid to. They are not even allowed to look at their own fannies!

THE LEGION OF THE DAMNED
A STORY OF PHYSICAL AND MENTAL AGGRESSION

This imaginary experience was not a fantasy but something based in physical reality; both the image and the realization of it came together in a combination of subjective and objective factors.

Men who join the Foreign Legion are men who have nothing to lose. When I said I had nothing to lose, I meant that I had lost all self- respect. At the age of ten, I was confronted by puberty, i.e. masturbation, and so appalled was I at this practice of self-abuse that, accordingly, I lost all respect for myself. By the age of fifteen this disgust had been increased by the actual sexual fantasies produced by adolescence, and I believed that my future relations with women would forever be denied to me; a year or so later I resolved to join the Foreign Legion to salvage my honour. By that time I was literally nothing but a fighting-machine, partly from the necessity of fighting for every breath I took, which I still have to today, and also for every movement I made. At one time it was all I could do to lift my little finger. I was probably fighting, also, against myself for the imposition of this disastrous condemnation, it having arisen, of course, by my own volition. My life since then has been the expression of an incredible aggression, that being the sole means by which I have been able to survive. However, the only redemption I might have had was thwarted by my very physical condition, which was so bad that at the age of nineteen I presented myself to a psychiatrist in a desperately suicidal state, having passed the whole of my time as a teenager fighting a losing battle.

One's sole purpose on earth, as you know, is to fight and to fuck; consequently, if you take away fucking – or the respect for woman – you lose your own self-respect – your only reason, basically, for living. The only thing you have left is your ability to fight; this becomes your driving force. I was driven to join the Foreign Legion in the single-minded determination to fight, and fight again; if necessary, to go down fighting – and very probably to die fighting; not in order to prove something, <u>but simply for the sake of it.</u> If the world had taken everything else away, at least it couldn't take that. You're in there to fight, and by God, that's the only salvation you have!

The Legion of the Damned was precisely that.

Dishing out punishment, I proceed through the corridors of life determined to put down all those who are falsely inclined; this obviously puts me in a dubious position inside a mental hospital! My physical appearance would not indicate it because, since the age of fifteen, though I have grown two inches in height, I haven't put on any breadth – in fact, since I was twenty, I have actually shrunk about two inches! (At that time, I was 5'11").

I conduct this purely on a verbal basis, because never in my life have I allowed myself to hit anyone, despite the fact that I have been in the ring quite a few times, and have had so many fights I can't remember; these have always been forced on me. You have to understand that, at the age of fifteen, I had to prove, <u>to myself</u>, that I was capable of standing up in a ring and having the shit knocked out of me without retaliating. Obviously I had to retaliate occasionally, to the dismay of my opponents, but for the most part my defensive powers were pretty ineffectual.

<u>You can only understand this restraint on my part if you acknowledge my identity...</u>

You might assume from my sexual experiences that I suffered from religious mania; not so. My experiences were self-inflicted, i.e. by my own will. Religious mania is usually imposed from without, by way of the irate father, or a vicar, or something threatening; sometimes it comes from the influence of the Bible, inoffensive in itself, though it is.

My 'religious mania' was actually my remit on earth: the requirement to be the most moral man in existence. Hence my dismay on being accused of any impropriety, whether sexual or otherwise, and particularly on being charged, as lately, with writing 'obscene letters'! – a thing which I have never done in my life.

An Early Love Affair

(I address all those who have accused me of lust)

It was while in this quandary that I first met Ella, and having been on the verge of suicide for a long time, I was suddenly provided with a reason for living. She made me idyllically happy for the next year, even though, at first, I could only regard her from a distance. For the first six months, I don't think anything happened, but this whole episode resolved my emotional crises vis-à-vis women. The paradoxical situation was this: even though my sexual fantasies had been, on the one hand, pretty objectionable – particularly to myself – I was at the same time in possession of the most mature and passionate dreams that could ever have been devoted to woman: pure and unadulterated – though sexual – love. These objectionable fantasies were, as I now realize, the direct expression of an insane desire to destroy myself; they had, in fact, nothing to do with sex, and, indeed, I never once inflicted them on Ella – nor have I ever defiled any woman in my life – including prostitutes: even though I was maniacally tempted, I always restrained myself in the knowledge that even a whore is still a woman; and therefore I did not expect the vilest creature to draw out of me what was in fact my only means of expression. So I was doubly crucified on this score alone, having remained in a state of suspension, generally, since the age of fifteen, and being subjected to it, without a moment's remission, for the rest of my life. This, I may say, is true self-control – if I have no other quality.

<u>There is, in fact, no sex in me whatever, and never has been.</u> What people have regarded as 'sexual frustration', was actually the instinctive expression of a protest at my physical condition, which was so extreme <u>that I had no expression at all,</u> except a very slight tendency to something which may have appeared sexual in origin but which was in reality caused by <u>a devastating anxiety</u>; the result of both my physical debility and my mental identity-crisis. This tendency was towards an habitual 'sexual' awareness, manifested partly in the genitals, causing a very minor irritation in that region. It most certainly was not an erection, or anything like it, though it was exacerbated by my constant need to urinate – a manifestation of anxiety in itself.

However, this irritation only contributed in a minor way, and infrequently, to my habitual walking impediment – a mental imposition – but this added 'peculiarity', however slight it was, caused ridicule wherever I went – not in itself, but, when combined with my undoubted inability to walk anyway, the two afflictions produced the most ridiculous appearance; and so, for this reason among many others, I have earned the title, 'The Idiot' – a figure, in a book by Dostoyevsky, who was depicted as Christ. Dostoyevsky, among others, was my prophet, the first being Wagner, in his prediction of the 'Perfect Man', the last being C.G. Jung, who forecast the 'Second Coming', due to take place at around the time of his own death. Which is what happened.

Almost exactly two years after Jung's death, I presented myself at the door of three Jungian analysts, who took one look at me and said, 'This is the man we've been waiting for'. They knew at once, yet no psychiatrist since has bestowed a glance on me – so taken up have they been with their own impenetrable egos. Jungian psychoanalysts, while they have discarded their self-love long ago, have still retained their intelligence, in distinction to the Freudian variety who, as well as discarding God, discarded, at the same time, their basic wits.

At the time I was addressing myself to these psychoanalysts, on a daily basis, I lived with Ella in her husband's home, he being my cousin. The ensuing love-affair, because of its distinctly beautiful nature, though it was at the same time highly unconventional, succeeded in establishing in my mind a certain confidence and self- respect, which had previously been woefully lacking. My self- destructive tendencies continued, however, alongside it – though not performed on Ella. This duality was obviously hard to reconcile, and it pursued me most of my life, but Ella provided me with a focus which enabled me to endure it. The Legionnaire was thus welcomed home.

Primed in this manner, I shall continue:

When I first saw Ella, I thought, 'Fuck me, now there's a frustrated woman!' Frustrated through love, not sex; I knew that from the start. Her husband was an impotent old goat who had subjected her to starvation for thirty years; when I reached her she was fifty still with a lovely, though severe, face and with the miraculously- preserved figure of Aphrodite. So modest was she that she would not be photographed in her bathing suit, a one-piece garment that served to conceal her very considerable charms from the prying eye and perhaps she was reluctant to be photographed, also, because the sexual implications were so important to her: she would not let this secret out of the bag to anyone. Though rejected by her husband, she still retained her womanly commitment to him as the only possible man in her life, and therefore she would not let anyone see her plight, or the charms she still reserved for him.

Every day, I saw this <u>woman</u>, whom I adored – and loved more, even than my own self driven to an emotional crisis which usually resulted in a migraine-attack; this was her daily regime. Her husband, a doctor, was forced to inject her, daily, with some drug designed to relieve her extremity; it was not very effective. But this injection, delivered quite high up on the thigh was the only intimacy, or love, that Ella received from her husband, and so she welcomed his attentions.

While she was in this desperate condition, I first came to live in Ella's home. So, desperate myself with love for her, I knew I had to take some action.

Walking in the woods one day, we stopped by a gate; Ella was looking, in an abstracted fashion, into the distance, with myself standing beside her. Whether I knew the implications of what I was doing, I don't remember, but I was determined to show her somehow what I felt for her; so I very gently and circumspectly placed my hand on the small of her back. Now, that is a highly significant place, as I knew; for it is mid-way between the heart and the body – that is to say, the business-end of the body – and therefore indicated love and physical passion combined. By my action, therefore, I was saying, 'I love you more than anything in the world; if you are willing to let me take you, I will, but I would not force you under any circumstances'. This certainly got through to her, but I was not sure how conscious she was of it; unconsciously she was very well aware of it, and she knew my intentions from then on. She did not reject me, but I soon withdrew my hand, respecting her enough to be prepared for a lengthy courtship.

Once, in an attempt to tell Ella of my identity, in response to her remorseful complaint that she was too old for me, I said to her, 'You are as young as the day you were born, And I am as old as Eternity'.

Reluctantly she replied, 'You're quite a poetic boy, aren't you?' My first poetic sally had met with a lukewarm reception, and my identity certainly remained in doubt.

On another, most singular, occasion, she told me that when she passed her old family home, after half a life-time's absence, she suddenly burst into tears; obviously she had been overwhelmed by memories of a once roseate and happy childhood…

LOVE'S WAY

One afternoon, after a flaming row – caused, probably, by my own fear that she did not love me – she ran off into the sitting-room in tears, crying: 'How can you say that to the woman who worships you!'

She had always been in the habit, when feeling particularly unhappy – which was frequently – of sitting down at her beloved piano and playing her favourite, and usually heart-rending, tunes.

Realizing the enormity of what I had done, I hastened to her and, loving this woman with all the unreserved passion which only I know, I approached her from behind, my own tears flowing copiously, and very tenderly placed my hands over her breasts. I knew very well what would follow. She rose immediately, and, tears ceasing, she took me by the hand and guided me to the sofa, where both of us had every intention of expressing our long-pent-up feelings. And so we did. She took off her skirt, and lay back over my knees, in abandonment to my love; this was a woman who, though never having experienced love before, knew just what to do – and she had the right man to do it.

Unfortunately, I was not able to have intercourse with her (a lifetime's forbearance). So I did the only thing I could do, and pushed my hand up her pants; as I couldn't immediately find her Intimacy, she whispered, 'Further forward'. So I entered her, with my hand, and in the determination to give her the utmost pleasure, I shoved it right up as far as I could – right up to the top of her little womb. The effect was immediate and devastating. How could so uniquely responsive a woman resist such a thing – The one and only fantastic orgasm she had ever received; there, in my arms, her lifelong frustration was released.

It was the first time in her life she had received any pleasure – and certainly any love. And so intensely did I love her that, when I withdrew my hand I placed it in my mouth, receiving the evidence of her passion. This was <u>the ultimate demonstration,</u> to Ella, of my love, not causing me, in any way, a thrill or pleasurable sensation. Surely such overwhelming <u>commitment</u> to a woman was never witnessed? – Demonstrating finally, to her, that this was not pleasure, but God's love, come down to earth for her. And in love, nothing is forbidden, and nothing is shocking. Anyone who thinks this was not love, has my fist to deal with.

And so, even at that tender age, though it was the first time I had ever made love to a woman, I knew so well how to do it: an expert in love, guided by love itself.

There was a practice at that time, in both America and over here, between couples who wished to make love before marriage, without spoiling it by actual intercourse, of comforting each other by hand. It was on this basis that our affair was conducted, because never, during the whole course of my life, have I permitted myself the ultimate knowledge of woman. Not even Ella succeeded in drawing this out.

My affair with Ella lasted only a year, because, knowing, after all, that she belonged to another man, and that I was knocking her off in his own house, I was forced to terminate it out of respect for him.

After I had gone, she never knew love again.

I have remained silent all these years in consideration for her family; I ask them to forgive me for my relations with their Mother.

This is the truth about my dirty liaison.

BUT DARKNESS DESCENDED

This is the terrible thing: Ella, the most innocent woman in the world – the one, above all, most capable of love – was led, by these very qualities, into the clutches of whoredom. Owing to a lifetime of denial, and total absence of any nourishment whatever, her very capacity for love was starved into the expression of its very opposite; her desperation resulted in hatred – hatred probably directed at her husband originally, but turned inwards on herself. For without the ability to project your feelings onto the one you love – because it would destroy them – you have no recourse but to destroy yourself. And so Ella's boundless love for her husband became converted into the consumptive passion of a whore.

Yes, those two extreme qualities can be combined in the same person; how many times have I observed this? So it was with dismay that I saw this happening. Without going into distressing detail, I will just say that, long before I got to Ella, she had been destroyed – perverted, in fact; this remained unconscious to herself – and to me – until, several times, it was revealed in her 'less spiritual' approaches to me. I have, unfortunately with frequency, been witness to the appalling paradox right at the heart of woman's nature: the Whore co-exists with the Mother; the former unconscious, the latter, conscious.

In a woman's normal life, assuming she hasn't been seduced either by herself or by somebody else, the Whore and the Mother world together harmoniously; the one complements the other; pleasure itself, the Whore, works together with spirit itself, the Mother – to produce Love, the over-arching Third Element. Love consists of the combination of pleasure and spirit, <u>and as long as both of them remain within Love, they retain their innocence</u>. But once they step outside Love, they automatically lose that innocence; they become dissociated – dissociated from each other, and from Love itself. In a case of sensational sex, which is a comparatively rare occurrence, innocence is maintained by the presence of both opposites – spirit and pleasure – even though Love itself may not be present. This situation is only possible through the existence of Unity, <u>the unconscious condition in which the opposites. spirit and pleasure, are unified, or in identification.</u> In this state of identification, the opposites are totally innocent – <u>because no-one can tell the difference between them: the Knowledge of Good and Evil – or consciousness – has not set in.</u> This womb of unconsciousness is the birthplace of Adam and Eve – innocent man and woman, both possessed of the indistinguishable opposites; we have, on the one hand, Adam – the Father and the Rake – and on the other, Eve – the Mother and the Whore. But when Eve eats the apple – <u>offered not by the serpent, but by God himself, for this is his design for humanity</u> – lo-and-behold, all hell breaks loose. Eve and Adam saw that they were naked! Eve looked at her fanny, and Adam looked at his chopper, and together they exclaimed, 'We are evil! What will the Lord think of us!' But the Lord shook his head, and said, 'Think not that you are evil, think not that you are good: <u>think both together, at once</u>'.

At one stroke, the situation is restored. Innocence returns to Adam and Eve, the Knowledge of Good and Evil receives its twenty-first century update, and everything from now on will be hunky-dory! – Providing you accept Christ – sorry, Anthony Wakefield Hill – a most unlikely name, which isn't even aristocratic – but in the guise of this much- persecuted lunatic, Jesus has come again to teach you – and to take away your ego.

Removing the ego of every man, woman and child entails the restoration of innocence to the psyche as a whole. One of the ego's most negative contents is masturbatory fantasies; now, whether you are a teenager or a supposedly grown man or woman, you will be subject to fantasies on two levels; first, sexual fantasies, and second, self-aggrandizing fantasies – both of which add up to self- love, or ego itself; so if you dismiss ego, you dismiss self-love, and consequently masturbation and self-aggrandizement as well. Quite an achievement! And worth doing, because if you <u>don't</u> dismiss these egoic qualities, you are left without innocence, maturity and love; in other words, you remain an evil man. The greatest evil is self-deception, brought about by self-love. Love must be turned outward, away from the self, and by thus attaining maturity, we do away with masturbation on all levels.

Masturbation, a horrible word – Dr J should have known better – is defined in two ways: self-abuse, and auto-eroticism; imprisoned in his, or her, fantasies, the masturbator flogs his tom, or, in the case of a woman, rubs her fanny, day and night in an attempt to imprison the opposite sex with him in his own mind. Even in the role of a rapist or paedophile, actually engaged on the job, the masturbator doesn't know who he is fucking or whether he is fucking at all. The solitary masturbator, tucked up in his stinking bed, doesn't actually try to abuse another person, thereby becoming a criminal, but he does abuse himself <u>by committing the cardinal sin of self-deception.</u> Whatever else we do, we mustn't dc that: God says, if we are going to do any fucking, we must fuck the real thing; a sensible recommendation, because if we don't fuck the real thing, how are we to make babies and perpetuate the human race? A point to consider, remembering that God also told us, I believe in the Bible, to 'go forth and multiply!' Darwin took up the cry, though I think he rather missed the point as usual, by telling us that fucking was for the specific purpose of procreation. Now I don't agree with that, and nor does God; God once imparted to me, in one of our nightly conversations, that man was put on earth to love; procreation is all very well, and very necessary, but Darwin was customarily concerned with the reduction of all life, love and learning to the one factor of Function. Unfortunately that definition remains with us today, and the chief legacy of 'Darwinian Evolution' is twofold: we all go around shagging like rabbits, convinced that there is no such thing as love, and, if there were, there shouldn't be, and everyone, despite his initial disgust, receives with alacrity his wife's well-meant farts projected from the anal-presentation position. This is on the recommendation of Darwin's devoted follower, Dr W, who informs us that love, or in his case, sex, should be performed on the basis of Smell. His conclusion, apparently, results from his observation of the sexual antics of apes with diarrhoea: what better smell could you get than that? He went so far as to demonstrate his findings with clinical tests. One further note: it emerges from the mists of the nineteenth century, a particularly backward era, that one of Darwin's colleagues, possibly Nietzsche, has apparently subtracted God from the universe; now, last time I saw him, about six months ago, the old boy was still alive and kicking, and he will be most surprised to learn that he is dead.

There is a grey area between the conscious and unconscious, generally known as the 'sub-conscious'; this is where the transactions between the unconscious, or Instinct, and the conscious, or Ego, take place; <u>obviously a very important area, and the relationship between Ego and Instinct has to be maintained, otherwise Ego becomes egotism.</u> The Ego itself is simply the area of consciousness: the consciousness of Self, or I. The normal consciousness of Self enables us to lead a civilized and harmonious life; although the Self actually includes the whole of the psyche, apart from the very grey area at the bottom of Instinct, where it is joined to the Universal Psyche, the actual consciousness of Self, or 'self-consciousness', is basically restricted to the egoic area. The remaining 'awareness' of self, probably moving to 'self-respect' in this regard, is essentially unconscious, manifesting itself emotionally.

It is this area, or aspect, of the psyche which has been under threat from psychology for over one hundred years; the very discipline set up to defend the mind's integrity, is responsible for its demise. This loss of self-respect, giving way to self-love, breaks up not just the sanctity of the psyche but also its wholeness.

THE CHEMIST'S SHOP

A girl I had known for some time, came to me one day and demanded that I love her. She and I had always 'felt' for each other. She was very warm and attractive, despite the fact that she wasn't obviously beautiful, and had a caste in one eye; but she was one of those unfortunate souls who had never found solace in her husband; now it was time I did something about it.

And so I made love to her – right there, on the spot, in that very chemist's shop.

We embraced. Taking her knickers down (always a prerequisite) without any circumspection whatever, I resolved to give her, once and for all, such love and passion as only Christ is capable of – with the greatest possible pleasure. With all my abundant masculinity, I reduced her to a fullness of swooning delight, and we eventually came to each other so closely that we didn't know who was whom.

'You darling, wonderful girl!' I managed to impart.

'You darling, wonderful man!' she whispered, just as she went under.

And I went with her, of course: that was the whole point of it.

Half an hour later, duty done, I said goodbye to her: 'You know, don't you, that this can never happen again? You have to go back to your husband'. 'Yes, I know'.

————————————

There is as much of a lobby against pleasure as for it. I favour neither point of view, but both.

————————————

Not only is pleasure an illusion, <u>but sex itself is an illusion</u>, sex being pleasure. The whole concept of 'sex' – and that means, expressly, not love – was born, latterly, of the late nineteenth-century notion that humans are naturally pigs; that is the unspoken, and underlying, implication if not the conscious admission. Darwin was almost singlehandedly responsible for it, his theory, 'The Origin Of Species', serving only to prove that, right at the beginning of Creation, there was, in God's mind, the design to separate out the psychological functions. Where Darwin went wrong was in deciding that everything in evolution <u>was physical;</u> he acknowledges the existence of mind – presumably – but this has, apparently, no bearing on the serious conduct of life, being merely a bloody nuisance when we are attempting to prove the non-existence of God. God will take a lot of convincing that he is defunct. However, if Darwin says so, He is, and He cannot argue with that.

Consequently, if God has died, his values, presumably, have died with him. And that is precisely what has happened. God's two chief purposes for man – to Love and to Learn – have been dismissed by Darwin as 'old hat' and when you say something is 'old hat' it gives carte-blanche to people like Pankhurst and Freud to follow suit.

Unable to think on their own account, they take up the prevailing trend and, through the only quality they do possess, unbounded conceit, they blithely assert that, God being dead, us humans can do what we like: no-one to punish us – the very thought would be criminal. Hence, 'Human Rights', the 'Declaration Of The Rights Of Man', the 'Rights Of Women', and just about every 'right' left in the book – <u>except the right to Self-Respect.</u>

On Self-Respect hangs every value Gad has vouchsafed us; from Love to Learning, to the Pursuit of Happiness – which comes about through the other two. We may be entitled to <u>pursue</u> happiness, but we have no inalienable right to happiness itself, which, if we ever do attain it, depends on our own efforts and not on God's bounty. In the pursuit of happiness, then, the first requirement of ourselves is Self-Respect. Self-respect is demanded of us by God, and presented to us by God. The First Law – not the First Right – is, 'Citizen, respect thyself'. Through this Divine Ordination, we are enabled to proceed through life, distributing bountifulness wherever we go and charity to all and sundry, in the knowledge within our souls that anything you or I may do depends ultimately on one thing – <u>the contract between God and man: each to respect the other, and man to respect himself.</u>

Not even the Pope has the right to wank in public; only the Son of God can do that. And he would do it <u>out of his own perverted self- respect, which leads him, through love, to destroy himself – on a public cross.</u> You see the Son of Man in his extremity: to be or not to be.

For, by being himself, he is forced to condemn man; and rather than condemn the very thing he loves most, he chooses to condemn himself, and ends up in life-long, self-crucifixion, finally resulting in the ultimate degradation of masturbating in public (fortunately only once). Such is Christ's disgust with himself, at his own duty, that he wallows in the shit of the sewers rather than pick himself up and become the Slayer of Man's Ego. Such an access of madness is incomprehensible, unless you consider Christ's incredible love for His own world, and for that wretch, man, whom He created out of His own sweat and blood.

Thus crucified, he continues today.

As we were saying, upon the withdrawal of his self-respect – something subtracted by Darwin's authority – man has evolved since the nineteenth century on a course of destruction and self-degradation – for much the same reasons as Christ, except that He was inspired by His own will, whereas man in his weakness follows the common herd. This respect for ourselves is required to be abandoned by the tenets of the 'Origin of Species', whether Darwin realized the implications or not, and today the situation is so extreme that, on every street-corner we see prostitutes trading their wares, and drug-addicts plying their needles. Masturbation is rife across the board – and not just in the instance of sex; in the illusion of existence itself we see reflected the illusions of every man jack of us.

Just as existence as a whole is a vast illusion, so physicality, including the body itself, is also a fundamental chimera; sex, pleasure, and the whole carnal gamut are beyond the pale of any reality whatever, the only semblance they might have had being spurted into nowhere by the ejaculations of an equally spurious masturbatory fantasy.

The overwhelming superiority of the mind over the body means that the body accounts for only one per cent of the reality of sexuality, the further ninety-nine per cent being reserved for the mind. The heart itself probably accounts for one hundred per cent of the mind in any sexual experience; consequently, it is impossible to approach a woman sexually except through Love, conducting the whole experience, furthermore, on the <u>basis</u> of Love.

THE FEMALE GENITALS

Holiest of Holies, Mystery of Mysteries – so the female cunt, and its attendant foliage; woman's most welcoming intimacy – an invitation, to man, of the utmost privilege.

Seen objectively, neither the female nor the male genitals might possess the utmost beauty; but beauty is in the eye of the beholder – or in the eye of the lover. And seen objectively, again – in other words, as an object – the pubic hair is automatically dissociated from the rest of the body, from which it <u>would</u> receive its true identity and aesthetic acceptance.

I would die for the honour of approaching such a threshold, being drawn from the ends of the earth to this sacred, mystical shrine.

When I observe a woman's hips – not her backside – I see them in the context of the whole body; that way, they aren't exaggerated or dissociated. I glance from the corner of my eye, so as not to look directly – which would be another insult to her.

To Venus

I am going to induce in you the utmost possible
   pleasure -
For you, in you, with you.
I will raise your passion to its highest and most
   ecstatic expression;
I know how to do it. I will do it.
With the greatest attention to detail,
In every possible way,
I will deliberately transport you into the most extreme
   orgasm
You could possibly imagine or receive.
And you will love me so much
That you will cry out in your very passion –

Right then and there – on the spot
Absolutely abandoned to the will of your Master.
And so you, my Mistress,
Having called forth my unfailing requite,
Will then rapturously relax in the afterglow
Of a fantastic experience,
Your face suffused with a lovely pink flush,
And your eyes regarding me, in their delighted
    mistiness,
With all the love which only a woman like you can
    offer me.

———————————

And if anyone asks you, 'Was this pleasure?'
You can confidently answer them, 'No, this was
    Love'.

E— came down to Lancashire from Carlisle, confronting me in Dr G's consulting room with one object in mind: to dish the dirt on me with as much force and infamy as possible. It has been her fondest belief about me, since her youngest days, that I am weak, ineffectual – if not actually cowardly – highly-strung and, into the bargain, sexually inexperienced and inadequate. So, she appears in the consulting room, first of all to let it be known what a twerp I am, and secondly to add her weight to Dorothy's beef about me, which she supports without reservation, knowing, in fact, nothing about my situation with Dorothy – which Dorothy herself does her best to obscure.

Contrary to this negative attitude, E— does in fact entertain some little regard for me, as a painter, and as a nice chap – weak, but nice; this is her positive side, which she would do well to cultivate, otherwise her position would be untenable.

Her opening words are: 'Hugh and Anthony pursued B— across a field'. I remember that field, because during our walk across it, I told B— my life story, and, far from pursuing her across it, I did in fact walk side by side with that young woman; nor did Hugh 'pursue her across a field', because Hugh was not even there on that day, my Mother having driven me to B—'s house. Apart from that field, there was no other field where either Hugh or I could have pursued her. It turns out that the original story came from B— herself.

'Pursing a young woman across a field', of course, has only one implication…

During our short association, B— made four main approaches to come, the first being in her sitting-room:

After quite a nice dinner (in the dining-room) she lay down on the floor in front of me – I was in an armchair – her hand between her thighs, directly below the intimate area (and she was very well aware of what she was indicating). This was our first date together, and such an invitation – obviously without love, or even spirit — was inappropriate, and unacceptable to a man like myself. This demonstration, which I had met with before from other women, did not fail to impress itself on me, although for her sake I pretended to be unaware of it (I find this the best response) feigning idiocy.

I could not get out quickly enough.

(B—'s sister, I am afraid – an actress, of sorts, and a mental patient – was the evil influence in this sororial relationship – full of pimples and under psychiatry's constraint: 'Get rid of the Mother at all costs' – the eternal cry).

This girl is of course an example of the powerful effect that a persuasive society can have on us, her present matronly appearance bespeaking years of sexual overstuffing – the direct result of the erotic expertise as expressed by psychology.

I hope B—'s husband didn't suffer the same approaches, of which I shall describe only one other:

In front of myself and a group of workmen, she made as if to climb over a gate, though she paused half-way over, her fanny resting on the top bar, though it must have been uncomfortable. She remained in that position for some appreciable time. 'What do you think those men were looking at?' she said afterwards. Like most men, they were probably looking at the fanny on offer – which I wasn't, to B—'s disdain.

So, once again the genital orientation raises its ugly head, totally dissociating sex from the rest of the body, thus forcing the isolated parts to endure a traumatic and exaggerated orgasm – Freud being the principal, though perhaps unconscious, authority to whom we are indebted for the genital-sex syndrome. Also dragging sex from spirit, tits from arse, and heart from head, he leaves the body finally dismembered and the mind deranged.

All this ends up making something dirty out of a woman's body – which God designed with the utmost respect – and something even dirtier out of a woman's mind.

Note To All Teenagers: Why You Can't Make Love

The reason you can't make love is that you are a mangy juvenile; you are immature: that is why you are a teenager. Teenagers can not have sexual intercourse because they have not grown up yet; the ability to achieve an orgasm is not an indication of man's estate. They haven't climbed out of the cradle yet, and don't know whether to put it in her ear or up her arse, which is the main reason why most girls don't get pregnant. If you were to put it up her vagina, you would ring the bell at once; consequently it is only the more intelligent who get pregnant – which isn't saying much. The rest of you are certainly wise enough to avoid the complications of love – if you know what that means.

But the complications of love, and growing up in general, are something you are unable to grasp; teenagers are not designed to make love until they have reached the stage of adulthood; and while they are still in their nappies, which is usually until the age of twenty or so, they are obliged to masturbate.

Wanking is the name of the game, and you must continue to wank yourselves silly until you are man enough to <u>Love</u>. For only Love will save you. And sex is made not <u>with</u> Love, but <u>for</u> Love, and <u>By</u> Love and <u>within</u> Love.

Remember that, all ye would-be Lotharios.

The Iniquity of the Rights of Man

THE CAUSE

DECLARATION OF INDEPENDENCE
(THE DISASTROUS FALL OF MAN FROM INNOCENCE)

The 1776 Declaration of Independence forced on us the notion of the right to rebel in defence of freedom, and a governmental system based on a 'natural law' involving 'the rights of the individual'.

Being a pragmatist, and nothing more, I point to this document as the most calamitously devised in modern history – responsible, as it is, for war upon war and revolution after revolution. <u>For it is based on a complete lie: that man has rights.</u> Quite apart from the fact that no American has ever known what an 'individual' is, no American has even known what a 'right' is, and certainly not what 'freedom' is. In order to obtain 'freedom', one has first to establish whether there is such a thing as freedom and what that freedom consists of.

Individuality, rights and freedom can be lumped together under the dictum: 'Individuality confers rights and freedom on itself'. Therefore, to have any freedom or rights, one has first to possess individuality, which is won after a lifetime's battle with oneself, and finally confers the right, and freedom, to think. It is not affected by any outside, or political, agency. Other than the ability to think, there is no right known to man.

Such political 'individuality' as exists is a mere numerative denomination, and, far from being individual, it is in fact profoundly collective and unconscious. Americans are, more than any other race in the civilized world, the least able to think. The only thing they are clever at is 'making a fast buck'.

This manifesto was fostered by the illusion that God himself has endowed man with rights: God never intended man to have any rights whatever – those being regarded as something which we can demand, on the basis that humanity is entitled to hold Creation to ransom. Creation in fact makes it quite clear that, as there are many essential processes in the world, they cannot be usurped by the application of rights to suit man's convenience, and that under no circumstances can evolution's laws be interfered with. Whatever claims man may make upon the powers that be, for the direction of society, <u>he must realize that this direction is already in place under the charge of evolution itself.</u> The promotion of the common man over the greater direction of society – already underway – is insupportable and wrong; man-made laws are neither ordained by Nature, nor inalienable, nor in any way binding on whatever authority gets in their way.

The Rights of Man are in no way inevitable or obligatory, and can not be imposed universally or indiscriminately. There are countries in the world who refute these laws, precisely because they are imposed without consideration for the very many exceptions to the rule; in fact there are so many exceptions that, in the Asiatic half of the world, the opposite is the natural law. In these countries, the introduction of Rights would jeopardize a perfectly viable social system and would be completely disruptive to a differing psychological background.

The idea, implicit – or explicit – in the Declaration, that Rights should be applied to everyone and everything right across the board, is in fact a dictation of the very sort that the document was designed to prevent. And in case you think that America couldn't be so unreasonable, just cock your ears to what Bush is declaring and ranting about incessantly.

The peasants were peasants because they had no intelligence; they were not 'born' to their lowly estate. Nor were they 'kept down'; they simply did not have the aptitude to climb up: exactly the situation which the 'Rights Of Man' was designed to perpetuate.

The conception of 'freedom', so prized in America, was apparently founded on the belief that everyone in the world, except Americans, was living under tyranny: 'Come to the land of the free': freedom from what, may I ask? I always understood that Britain herself, from whom the U.S.A. sought to part company, so prized her own freedom that she fought against Napoleon – not to mention the Kaiser and Hitler – to prove that point.

Man's freedom may be a desirable thing, but man does not have a right to it, and certainly not the right to demand it. In fact, the 'natural' freedom of man does not even exist, and can never exist; the only freedom granted by God to man, apart from the capacity to think, is to die – and even that is taken away from us by 'civil liberties'.

The USA's undying intention is to impose freedom on everyone and everything else, regardless of circumstances and with unlimited powers to dictate its acceptance. Americans have to take a tumble to themselves, and to realize that their nation was founded on a complete chimera. Hard as it may be to believe, and contrary to all viciously-held traditions in America, this fact has to be acknowledged and accepted; otherwise there is no hope for world peace. The United States is the threat, not Russia or China.

There was no justification, of course, for Bin Laden's attack on New York, and America has every right to retaliate; which is why the war in Afghanistan, at least, is a just one. Fundamentalism is an evil which must be expurgated, but what Bin Laden is fighting against is not the illusion of freedom, but values held in the Western world which are inimical to all innocent ideas supporting the lives of decent and self-respecting people everywhere else. Offensive beliefs emanating from Europe and America did in fact provoke the '9/11' disaster. That they also provoked Bin Laden's own inferiority- complex is largely irrelevant, except that this sense of inferiority is widespread throughout the East and results not least from America's arrogance.

There are more wars caused by the actual idea of freedom than by any physical necessity for it, such is human susceptibility, and this unsubstantiated belief in the obligatory 'call to arms' has produced more wars since the Declaration Of Independence than at any previous time in history.

Contrary to the popular belief in the U.S.A. that Britain wielded tyrannical power over that fledgling country, the American Revolution was actually caused by the somewhat more insignificant attempt to impose taxes on the tea industry; apart from that, British rule was not objectionable, and was only thought to be so when George Washington managed to persuade his impressionable countrymen that rule from London was somehow undesirable; and being imbued with the notion that both his and his country's destinies were bound up, he came to the irresistible conclusion that he had been chosen – by someone unspecified – to conduct a war against what would normally be considered a rather reasonable regime. But there you are: George never told a lie, did he?

The idea that the United States was preternaturally destined to lead the 'warriors of freedom' in a holy war against all and sundry, was both the cause and the result of that country's totally unfounded assumption that God had his eye on the American people. How they knew that, I don't know, because God never told me anything of the sort, and I was under the impression that I was here to prove exactly the opposite. So one of us has to go. I will definitely be crucified – there is no doubt about that – and the Americans are just the buggars to do it; if I dare set foot over there, I am sure Uncle Sam will set the dogs onto me. But that is a risk I have to take; the need to put down America's rampant ego is too important to be abandoned.

The world was not invented for the masses, and their leader, Christ, is an élitist. Existence is a gift awarded to those who are prepared to exert themselves, man's chief quality being, unfortunately, laziness. Therefore, an end to all revolutions, and the damnable right to life, liberty, and the pursuit of happiness, which can only be found in the service of others and the sacrifice of personal freedom.

America is founded on a lie – nay, a series of lies – and far from being the self-styled saviour of the world, it has been a primary source of world-suffering – unwitting to itself, maybe, but thereby all the more to be condemned. I bring Consciousness; and there is no greater enemy of man than the abysmal absence of that quality, which is the subliminal cause of the proposed imposition of rights and freedom in the first place. Unless the U.S.A. and the rest of the world realize the basic Lie at the root of man's condition, there is no hope of anyone attaining any freedom – freedom, that is, from the Lie itself. Other than the freedom of the conscious individual to think for himself, there is no freedom, and never was designed to be.

The only God-given right of man was indeed the God-given freedom of the enterprising citizen to meditate of his own volition; it was declared vociferously by Europeans hundreds of years ago, and not latterly by some insolent band of American Fathers.

The Lie at the root of man's condition is nothing less than the universal belief that 'I am as great as God'; and that is why man crucifies God – because he does in fact know the truth, and he can't accept it.

I bring the truth; I will be crucified.

In declaring man's entitlement to absolute freedom, and his absolute right to this, that and the other, man himself is setting himself up as God, for only God has the right to make such laws. Democracy, far from being a God-given sentiment, would, more accurately, be from the Devil, for, in its pursuit, there have been countless acts of mass violence.

George Bush, the clown at the helm of the Western World, was voted in on the basis of his nice smile and the public's willingness to overlook his obvious mental deficiency, these being his sole qualifications. This cowboy in jeans, who should have stayed mucking the pigs out on his ranch, has managed to con the West into accepting his version of the USA's perennial manifesto. By a combination of their leaders' egotism and their own unassailable naivetée – a distinguishing feature of these people – the citizens of America have been led into one state of confrontation after another, on the platform of the deluded proclamation that man has rights. From that alone there has issued a constant international tension, and the egos, both national and individual (and also the naivetée) of the warring countries have invariably been inflamed by the illusion that freedom – whatever that is – is obligatory to every self-respecting man; and despite the frightful consequences of, fratricidal conflict, brother has turned on brother, and both together have turned on what is more often than not an inoffensive and benign government. Shouting the odds against one and all, these macho heroes take a swipe at anything they suspect of having designs on their manhood – and the apparent oppression by any hapless government is enough to persuade them of that. Freedom in the name of manhood is the creed that inspires, and confuses, most primitive mentalities, which are unable to distinguish between the demands of egotism and a possible intellectual cause. Rousing the rabble is a vested interest of so-called intellectuals the world-over, and so much the better if it is based on a lie. This usually results in the confusion of the idea of maleness with the desire to 'throw off the yoke' – a cry which never fails to appeal to the tribal war-mongers, whether or not it is accompanied by a reason. From the jungles of Africa to the more sophisticated ale-houses of Edinburgh, the eternal incitement to take up arms is met with immediate enthusiasm; and even if, in the case of Edinburgh, the bearing of offensive weapons is not required, Scottish manhood rallies to the cause: 'Down with England! What have those buggars ever done for us! Ever since Robert the Bruce shuffled off this mortal coil, those English fuckers have levied taxes on our whisky, and stolen the salt from our porridge!' Alex Salmon, a stern representative of human rights and freedom – at least when it comes to Scotland – is particularly clamorous, though I have not, as yet, been able to perceive any reason for his rabid incantations against his historical neighbour. It is a bit out of date, wouldn't you say? Maybe two or three hundred years ago, it would have been appropriate to preach fire and brimstone against the English oppressor, but can you tell me exactly how England is oppressing him today?

Despite the civilization, i.e. the cultural and economic development, that Scotland has derived from the English, and which has rescued it from the hordes of kilted heathens, there has arisen in the misty North a belatedly dissenting voice which is determined to prove how superior in every way Scotland is to England. That this conviction emanates from Salmon's own overweening ego, and not by any means from the more modest disposition of the average Scottish clansman, is a fact yet to be rumbled by the slumbering natives both north and south of the border. The Declaration has worked its evil influence even amongst the sublimely unconscious peaks and valleys of our once-limited kingdom. The obvious necessity for unity in our troubled world is being deliberately obstructed by the call for liberty and privileges which is broadcast, universally and incessantly, with the aim of inspiring innocent people to rise up against what is misrepresented as 'oppression'. Countries such as Tibet and Burma, which genuinely do suffer from oppression, are in the very exceptional minority, being governed, unfortunately, by regimes which exhibit an infantile mentality and are subject to the most primitive beliefs. These nations have every excuse to use violence, but they are counselled, in the instance of Tibet, by the wise old Dalai Llama, who forbids violence under any circumstances. The Dalai Llama also counsels that Tibet should remain, whatever the outcome of the protest, under Chinese rule. This would, of course, provide the ideal solution, <u>as it would preserve an indispensable unity</u>. The Chinese may eventually bow to world opinion, <u>that having been inspired by the unarmed resistance, and peaceful protests, of the Tibetans.</u> What the Tibetans are seeking to achieve <u>is the freedom of the individual to conduct his own inward-looking meditation: in other words, the freedom to think.</u> This is the 'religion' that the Chinese are trying to suppress; <u>in a totalitarian state, a free-thinking individual poses threat: he questions its authority.</u>

And so it is, in the apparently free world of the West. We in the West use exactly the same tactics as the Chinese, to the same end; any society founded on the right of the establishment to impose the very suppression it is ostensibly designed to prevent, is in danger of succumbing to schizophrenia. The only way to save such a society <u>is to introduce freedom: the freedom of the individual to think.</u> Without thinking, society goes under.

America is as much the enemy as China (or Iran). Freedom is threatened by China on a physical basis, but America threatens the very freedom she professes to defend; man has only one freedom and that is to think for himself, and it is this, precisely, that America is attacking.

It is not only America's own ego that sparked off the '9/11' attack, but also the very aggression demonstrated by the U.S. in her 'declaration of intent'. This is a direct challenge to the ego, and obviously to the freedom as well, of other countries. <u>What we have here is the confrontation of egos, and the mutual threat to freedom. This is the classic cause of all wars.</u>

It is probably true that China threatens America on a purely physical basis, and that America threatens China on a mental basis, <u>since neither nation can actually think (as far as politicians are concerned)</u> and such intellectual freedom as they both have is extrovert on America's part and introvert on China's, these two psychological functions actually being the even more fundamental cause of the conflict, representing, as they do, the intellectual <u>character</u> of each party. On the one hand we have the individual nature of the Chinese mentality, on the other we have the collective nature of America's; <u>this has always been the underlying, and even more basic, cause of antagonism throughout world history.</u>

The only way this constant threat to world peace can be overcome <u>is by the conscious address of both the egoic and the psychological differences, realizing the actual identity of the two modes of thinking involved.</u>

Because China's psyche is basically introverted, her thinking function (confined to her intellectuals) <u>is conscious and therefore far more individual than America's</u>. America's psyche being basically extroverted, her thinking function <u>is unconscious and therefore essentially collective.</u> Because thinking, in China, is conscious and, in America, is unconscious, it follows that China's psyche is not only individual but also free, while America's is collective and therefore captive. Therefore America is defending her freedom – a purely physical devotion to a numerical individuality – <u>against a physical attack, while China feels her freedom threatened on a mental basis</u>; of the two, China's mental attitude is by far the more intelligent, and consequently America should seriously consider whether her freedom is actually as valuable as her enemy's: the freedom to do no more than eat, sleep and fart can hardly be compared to the habitual application of metaphysics.

The difference between the two egos is apportioned on a similar basis. We have, on the one hand, the introverted inferiority complex of Asia and, on the other, the extroverted superiority complex of the West. They complement each other: the schizophrenic division between the world's hemispheres, neither being aware of the other's true existence, each tearing the other' throat out as a consequence. As far as egotism is concerned neither is superior, China's initial inferiority giving rise to her desire for superiority – in all things, from territorial conquest to the possession of the atom bomb – America's <u>resultant</u> superiority arising from her <u>initial</u> inferiority – that arising from the Occidental; self-comparison with God himself, purely unconsciously. These are facts which it is very easy to prove: the underlying reality; man is a Savage Beast. Why has God come to earth at this time?

The intellectual life of China is, or was before Mao Tse Tung, far more advanced than that of the U.S., and also on a far wider scale, being present particularly in Buddhist monasteries, Buddhism being not so much a religion as a philosophy; in comparison, America's intellect is non-existent.

Peace is founded on negotiation, not on the threat to drop bombs on everyone who opposes you. It is this very threat, carried out by the U.S.A. not only in the past but also right now, which is largely responsible for the hostile reactions of Muslims and the rest of the world generally. It is directly responsible for the war in Iraq, for which there was not any viable reason, never mind an excuse, except for America's habitual bellicosity and bloody-mindedness. A minimum of diplomacy backs up the underlying desire to solve everything by force.

<u>Bush and Blair were itching to flex their muscle – what Prime Minister wouldn't? – and despite the predictable denial, this was the unconscious and ultimate purpose of their being in power: to save the country – by flattening any aggressor; what are all those planes and ships waiting for? Go on! – this is the ultimate test of your manhood! Push the button!</u>

The annihilation of Iraq was brought about by the monstrous ego of America, and Tony Blair, which persuaded them, against the promptings of reality, to bomb the bloody shit out of the place. Despite Tony Blair's assumption that he is a reasonable and peaceful man, this restrained approach did not prevent him, without needing much persuasion, from unleashing the holocaust, Saddam' personal proclivities being dragged in afterwards as an excuse.

How, by any stretch of the imagination, could Saddam

possibly have attacked either England or America in their homelands? And if this whole campaign was conducted on the basis that we were stepping in to pre-empt a possible conflict somewhere in the Middle East (a comparatively small area) – another professed motive – why would we need to get our knickers in a twist over that? The 'World Policeman' retired long ago; NATO wouldn't take a hand for the same reason.

The American military, of course, as ever, could not wait to go into action to show those cowardly Iraqis just how brave and tough the American 'fighting man' is; and that is the sole motive for the American soldier's decision to join the army – to prove to the world that he is 'top dog' and that everyone else is a quaking poltroon – demonstrated in every war film and best-seller, and shouted to the rooftops by the nation's own habitual attitude, bristling with aggression and mean intent. The truth, as usual, will be denied, because ego itself blinds us to it.

The whole creed on which the American nation was founded, and its subsequent traumatizing effect on the rest of the planet, was based on a criminal misrepresentation; and this fact, which will be furiously rejected, has led to the belief on the part of its citizens that their country was set up by God to represent man's right to absolute freedom. The very fact that they will under no circumstances withdraw this conviction, will undoubtedly plunge the world into even deeper chaos, as we are seeing today in Iraq, and furthermore in the USA's declared intention to reduce Iran, also, to rubble.

There was in fact no negotiation between the Allies and Saddam; such sanctions as there were, had been put in place long before to topple a repressive regime, and this idea was only trotted out as the excuse for the invasion when it was discovered belatedly that there were no weapons of mass-destruction after all. Having his justification taken away from him, what did Blair do but play the card of 'regime-change', when, previously, it had not 'figured'? No doubt convincing even himself, Tony managed to fudge the issue so that a not-too-observant public was also convinced. The 'toppling of the tyrant' became the government's very popular order of the day; amongst all the furore, who now remembers 'weapons of mass-destruction'?

We offered Saddam no chance to adjust his position vis-à-vis W.M.D., and even if these elusive weapons had been found, they could have posed no threat at all to the safety of the West. But Bush and Blair's chronic sense of insecurity convinced them, apparently, that Iraq's rockets were aimed directly at their own countries, thousands of miles away; by their own admission, the rockets in question could not reach further than Israel, so unless we are to assume that the whole war was conducted in defence of Israel (which wouldn't surprise me) we are faced with the inescapable conclusion, which has received confirmation many times before, that Bush and Blair are a couple of schizophrenics, manifesting the whole delusional, paranoid and anxiety-ridden syndrome, exacerbated by its totally unconscious character. And think not that apparently 'normal' people are innocent of this crippling disease; politicians are ones who are constantly struggling to keep it at bay, and as far as Iraq and Tony Blair are concerned, it seems to have got the upper hand. If Blair had been premier of Germany in World War II, he would have acted in the same way, but as he is premier of Britain today, he gets away with it. Of course, this won't worry him – his ego's too thick.

If the rockets could not proceed beyond Israel, even I, who am not renowned for my mathematics, must ask, 'How could they reach America and Britain?' This glaringly obvious question has never been asked before, and certainly never answered. The only alternative cause for the two stooges' insecurity complex, is the even wilder reasoning that, in some way, a war involving Iraq would spell automatic disaster for our two countries – again contrary to the logical question, 'Aren't we two thousand miles away?' Even by endowing the two leaders with commonsense, one couldn't credit their belief that a Middle-Eastern embroglio would seriously jeopardize the safety of Britain and America, whether directly or indirectly – unless some raving Iranian mullah were inspired to call down the wrath of God on the decadent West – which appears to be the case, since Marks and Spencer were recently stunned to learn that they had lost the contract to supply cheap clothing to the Arabs. Unprecedented disasters such as this, the result of a Middle- Eastern embargo, would seem after all to justify our leaders' fears!

But, seriously, I fully expect Blair to try and wriggle out of this one by claiming that all these motives were his policies: a mixture – and a fine potpourri at that! These policies can in fact only work together if you discount the facts about them individually; in other words they can't be combined – so sort the bones out of that.

The absolute refusal of the United States to even consider that its basic premise could be wrong, presents the world with an insoluble problem; not only are the Western leaders subject to schizophrenia – even being unaware that their policies are hopelessly contradictory and inconsistent – but they are also incapable of thinking logically, which is actually consistent with the illness. But on no account would Blair admit this; Bush might, because his mental capacity leaves him open to the persuasion that 'all good men admit their faults'.

But between the two of them they manage to present a united front, thus lending stability to an otherwise unstable mental condition; if you are convinced that you are a messiah – another thing Blair is unconscious of – you may very well decide to dispense with all reason and substitute your gut-feelings in every way possible; and because Blair is a quasi-Communist, nevertheless managing to conduct an illicit affair with Conservatism, his gut- feelings tell him to fool the world into thinking he is both. This, of course, is impossible because, as we know, Labour and Conservative would never be seen in bed together; but in Blair's mind there is no distinction between Red and Blue, and also no distinction between truth and falsehood.

In accord with the convolutions of the schizophrenic mentality, Blair's situation is understandable: on the one hand he convinces himself that he is Red, on the other hand he convinces himself that he is Blue; but where he falls down is in trying to convince himself, also, <u>that he is both at the same time</u>. Not even a schizophrenic can do that. The pathological mind is polarized; in other words, you can't have your cake and eat it at the same time. The trouble with Blair is that he doesn't know whether he's got his cake in the first place, or how to bloody well eat it anyway.

So it should be evident by now that our Prime Minister is in no position to pass judgment on world affairs (Substitute Brown for Blair).

Once the Americans had scented blood, nothing could stop them. What in fact scented the blood, was not so much their noses as their insane egos. <u>Ego is a fact, and never more so than in America; it drives the economy, it drives the government, it drives the psyche.</u> This nation, boasted to be the champion of the free world, is so governed by egotism that it cannot see its own infamy; and rather than admit the screamingly obvious truth, it sends envoys around the world charged with persuading everyone that this belligerent hive of conceit is their best friend; read it in America's eyes, read it in America's face, read it in America's brutally arrogant behaviour – which it doesn't even attempt to disguise, so convinced is it that God is on its side.

This must be said; this must be believed; otherwise the U.S.A. will continue to trample on all who get in her way. Her self-belief is <u>beyond</u> belief, her blindness to herself is only surpassed by her blindness to others.

The original Declaration was inspired by the baseless conception of 'God's Own Country' – notwithstanding that identical assumption on the part of many other nations. All this was compounded by the ego of the average citizen, which was in turn fostered by a rather mysterious thing, in far-off Europe, called the 'Social Contract'. Whatever the original meaning, or purpose, of this contract, it took root in the U.S.A. as the subliminal relationship between the ego of the private citizen and the even more overwhelming ego of the nation as a whole – represented, of course, by the 'American Fathers' themselves. All the egoic strands of this relationship – that is, the individual citizens – were held together and facilitated by what I have described as 'the collective confidence-trick' – a process of mutual blackmail: 'You scratch my back and I'll scratch yours – but woe betide you if you don't'. Present in most countries of the world, the mutual confidence-trick is, and was at that time, modified by the very process it entails; for in its intention to subdue all genuinely 'individual' resistance, it solidifies and draws together the membership of society as a whole, so providing it with an essential unity. <u>The fabric of civilisation is therefore based on its</u>

own warp and woof: the intricate interweaving, and interlocking, of its many egoic parts.

Individual resistance obviously has to be suppressed because, by thinking, the individual sees the gaping flaws in society's structure – and in those days he was burnt at the stake for doing so. However, the diabolical process of suppression, nowadays, takes place on a more insidious basis; but, put in a nutshell, it would proceed like this: 'You keep my ego going, and I'll keep yours going, and together we'll keep society's going'. And let me tell you that there is nothing more truly diabolical than Egoic Man – both towards himself and towards others.

THE INFAMOUS DECLARATION

The only right man has, is to become himself through thinking. He certainly has no right to assert himself, and still less right to expect any rights.

God put us on earth for his own purposes, meaning that we are here on sufferance; we are God's retainers, and retainers have no rights except to be retained. God's dispensation can not be thrown back in his face by a demonstration of tantrums, designed to compel him to withdraw his intentions.

The most destructive event of modern times was America's misconceived Declaration of sundry rights; this unfortunate occurrence has had the most dire consequences for mankind ever since, causing endless wars and presenting us, on the home front, with Womens' Rights and the Feminist Movement – all with the one intention of defying God's purpose for man; which is, to have no rights at all. In defying God's most basic law, America has introduced chaos onto earth, which we see constantly around us in the demands, on every possible occasion and against all reason, for 'life, liberty, and the pursuit of happiness'. Happiness will never be found in the arms of either life or liberty; life, or existence, is demonstrably an illusion, and liberty has yet to be proved desirable. The assumption that any of these three qualities is either necessary or desirable is unwarranted and has never been substantiated. Far to the contrary, our subsequent history has proved exactly the opposite. The world would not be in the mess we see today if Thomas Jefferson had not been drunk on the

Fourth of July; only a befuddled mind could have produced such a fallacious idea. His intellectual qualifications were not inspiring, consisting of a knowledge of the bible and a few philosophical persuasions culled from other peoples' concepts – and not much else. Along with a few other unqualified pundits he has managed to convince the 'free' world that freedom – if there actually is such a thing – is worth fighting for – indeed, that it is obligatory to fight for it. First of all, the true nature of freedom has never been revealed to the world – I am bringing it for the first time – and secondly, it is doubtful that two catastrophic world wars have actually proved that fifty million dead people mean it was worth it. That the 'free world' remains is due not so much to the fighting capacities of the American solider as to the fact that the few hundred million survivors avoided extinction.

Freedom, therefore, as defined by Thomas Jefferson, has proved to cause more misery and suffering than it was intended to prevent. Is it actually worth fighting for?

I like fighting, myself, but I have yet to meet the grieving mother who thought the sacrifice of her son was worth the blood and gore that produced it. The American soldier's attempt to prove how heroic he is – constantly thrust in our faces by John Wayne – is the underlying force behind his country's persistent determination to go to war. This all-consuming desire for 'heroism and sacrifice', in the service of an illusionary freedom, stems from the same disastrous, romantic fantasy that produced the 'Declaration' in the first place.

Western culture has developed, despite itself, an obsession with personal freedom. This very obsession has produced exactly the opposite result to that which it was initially intended to procure: it has ended personal freedom. Every Western society is now a totalitarian state. That is not an exaggeration; it is not an extreme statement. I wish it were.

You, the Western citizen, have turned yourself inside out; black has become white, white has become black. Good has become evil: exaggerated good automatically becomes its

<u>opposite.</u> And, in this case, the desire to introduce personal freedom has become exaggerated. The very safeguards to personal freedom have been removed, the chief of them being the ability to think; no-one can think if he is denied the facility to do so; that is, a thinking environment, or an environment conducive to thinking. When Tony Blair took it upon himself to abolish the grammar schools – evidently to disguise his own source of education, public schools being only one step removed – he destroyed the main educational facility of the working classes. This hypocritical attempt to do away with his past – in fact to betray his own origins – was designed to prove to the working classes that 'he was one of them'. And what better could you have than that? – Betray your own lineage, and the world is yours.

But in attempting to prove this to the working man, Blair in fact removed the very source of the working man's education. By everyone's admission, grammar schools had provided the best, and only, route that the working man could take in order to reach success. And now where are they? They have been replaced by all sorts of queer establishments, culminating in something called an 'academy'; and as far as I can make out, these 'academies' are actually no different to the original grammar schools. Apart from their different name, they serve exactly the same purpose – which is, if I am not mistaken, 'higher education' (or is it 'further education'?) But of course, the original purpose of abolishing grammar schools, apart from Blair's disguise, was to deprive the working man of 'higher education' – otherwise, why abolish them? Now, the working man has been got in by the back door so that we won't know he is receiving 'higher education' – or so I must assume, because by now I am beginning to realize that the Labour Government, as well as being deceitful, is also very probably schizophrenic. If you can figure out the desperate convolutions, contradictions, withdrawals and re-instatements sent, evidently, to reduce the educational system to chaos, you are a better man than I am – and I shall retire to a rest home.

But the secret is out. Don't I hear you telling me that the real reason why grammar schools were abolished was the intention <u>to make everybody equal?</u> Well, I am sorry to inform you that no-one on earth can make everyone else on earth equal; that is God's job and he says that under no circumstances should everyone be equal – that in fact it is impossible for everyone to be equal: are you as clever as I am? And if you are not, then you are not entitled, by all natural laws, to be educated to a higher level; you are simply not intelligent enough; the teachers would be wasting their time, and if by some fluke you ended up in a decent job, you would very soon be sacked. The world is for the intelligent: God says so, and, by all the laws of evolution, the success of this planet is based on 'the survival of the fittest' – not just when the monkeys were playing around, but also now when the contest is between minds. I could take two of you on and reduce you to mincemeat – which is why I have been selected by Nature to write this sermon.

Christ, the man sent to instruct this universe, is an élitist – and proud of it. Furthermore, he is a Conservative, and would have no truck with Labourites, or any other trogs, if he could possibly avoid it. Labour is based on 'equality for all', and even if you take that to mean 'equal opportunities', the whole idea is scuppered from the start by the inability of the common man to muster the intelligence for it. Equal opportunities are wasted opportunities, and if Labour insists on promoting the herd, let it not do so at the expense of those who are clever enough, and sufficiently motivated, to make their own way in the world; that means not holding them back, in schools and classes which are designed specifically for the mentally-deficient. Unfortunately, three-quarters of the population _is_ mentally-deficient, thus rendering it necessary to re-instate the grammar schools.

The Result

Deception In High Places
(How Democracy Is A Front For Man's Self-Deception)

Attention, all public relations wallahs! Ensconced as you are at the heart of public affairs, you must be aware that a more dishonourable occupation never slithered across the face of society.

Teaching your clients how to twist your neighbour, how to employ every dirty trick in the book, how to lie without being found out – this is how you proceed, despite your undoubted ability to remain oblivious of it. All this is calculated, and disguised so as to be acceptable to the more gullible of us, notwithstanding your efforts to present an innocent face, which is quite deliberate though unconscious.

The most degrading profession ever to disgrace the offices o1 business – or any other field – features as its cornerstone an invidious school of charm, which teaches one to dissemble without alerting the victim, and arms one with the confidence to cheat without the inconvenience of guilt – the modern trend being to approach life from the point of view of total cynicism, no genuine feelings being allowed in this world of sophistication, where any suggestion of innocence is dismissed as immature. This, of course doesn't matter, because everyone in society subscribes to the assumption that life is a charade and that therefore we are entitled – even obliged – to conduct ourselves on a spurious and shallow basis; the more people we take in, the more sophisticated we are considered to be. This is the unspoken, yet underlying reality of contemporary psychology.

The cultivation of deliberate artifice is now expressly taught in our universities, and schools of 'self-development', the latter having mushroomed ever since the Hollywood Attitude displaced the commonsense of our more impressionable citizens.

And if you don't recognize this as yourself, your capacity for self- deception equals your capacity for deceiving others.

Such are the credentials of the brigade of public relations officers lately recruited into politics, as the advisory experts in the background; these advisors have reduced the government to a body of shysters intent on misleading the country at every turn. Exaggerated, you say: here again, if you don't believe what I am saying, you should take a closer look at yourself – under that calculated front. The smug, angelic, self-satisfied smiles of the Labour front-bench spokeswomen say everything that needs to be said about the true face of the cabinet. Their holier-than-thou, sanctimonious assumption that they, and only they, are right – on every question – and could not be otherwise, sickens all those with an objective viewpoint. You may not think that this bears particular significance, but let me assure you that this very assumption of theirs belies their apparent innocence; an innocence that is actually the most destructive and deceptive part of their make-up; for it is deliberately intended to disguise the iron fist in the velvet glove. These very attractive women, in whose mouths butter wouldn't melt, are in reality the hellions behind Labour's collective Ego – and Ego, let me say, supersedes even innocence as the most destructive part of their psychology, being the very thing which innocence is at such pains to disguise. Who said that women didn't have ego? – Particularly women in high places?

Their evident belief that the Labour government was uniquely destined to lead the world into the promised land of innocence and plenty, where everyone would worship their political leaders as messiahs, is somewhat contradicted by the unfortunate truth: that Labour's pristine virtue is sullied by the illusion that divine right confers on them an exemption from all criticism, which they roundly and habitually dismiss with a wave of their intolerant hand.

They will deny this of course; they wouldn't want to think that their dainty little hand would tamper with the process of truth… such delicate, lady-like behaviour as they exhibit in the service of the welfare state could not possibly be contaminated by unladylike egotism – that snake which lurks just beneath the surface of our so- placid lives.

The grey iniquity of Gordon Brown himself may be unwitting, but it is all the more redolent of Lucifer for that; the more inoffensive and plausible we seem, you may be sure that we are the opposite underneath, the character of the primitive savage having remained unsubdued since primeval history – leading us into predatory behaviour even in the sacrosanct quarters of politics.

While maintaining his Presbyterian facade, Gordon Brown subliminally pursues a dangerous course of misrepresentation, designed to convince everyone that he is, on the one hand, the Angel Gabriel, doing as his Father demanded while he was a callow youth, and, on the other, that he and his ministers have nothing but the people at heart; whereas the fact is that they are occupied in milking the susceptibilities of a vulnerable electorate, to the extent of persuading them that everything in the Labour

Government's policies is not only hunky-dory but actually beyond any possibility of disagreement, and that their self-projected image is sacrosanct – 'and we dare you to question that'. There is none so blind as man to himself, and the Labour cabinet is no exception.

Incredible! Unacceptable! you cry. But look at you: are you in any position to judge? – You, who are so unaware of your <u>own</u> proclivities that you believe <u>yourself</u> to be sacrosanct? – beyond reproach even? So you are convinced when treading the corridors of power.

Where, actually, does the truth lie? The average politician, bereft as he is of the refinements of conscious living, is immersed, as we have said, in ego, unable to think in even the simplest terms – beyond the calculation of the daily bowel-movement – and so unconscious as not to know anything of significance; possessing, furthermore, so little will that his mind bows to the slightest mental pressure. This unfortunate automaton struts around Westminster just as if he had the right to be there, which indeed he wouldn't have if his true mental capacity were suspected. He furthermore exhibits the characteristics of a quivering jelly in the face of physical opposition; rather than hit somebody in retaliation for being attacked, he would actually resort to suing them in court. And he leads our country?

All in all, we are represented by a gang of self-serving opportunists – in contradistinction to their own, self-deluding belief: a case of the blind leading the blind.

This is a portrait of the human being: if you do not recognize yourself, take heart from the monkey's inability to reflect on anything at all.

What do I think of Tony Blair? – a public relations expert, only surpassed in this regard by that arch-Machiavellian, Alistair Campbell, the author of 'New Labour': a scheme, as dishonest as its creator, which was designed to manipulate the public into accepting a few adventurers as the leaders of our country, with as few political qualifications as possible, and, further, to maintain them in power as long as they succeed in hoodwinking Parliament with diabolically clever speeches, learned from years of wheeling and dealing at the Bar. The Nineteen Ninety Seven –

election was fought and won on the basis of scurrilous allegations by New Labour – dug up by nocturnal investigations into the parliamentary dunghill – against those unfortunate members of the Tory Party who had dared to indulge in an extra-marital affair – which would not have excited a murmur if Blair and his cohorts had not been determined to drive them out – by fair means or foul. All fair politics? – Not in the hands of past-masters of smear and calumny campaigns. Yes, Tony, this is how you came to power; <u>you</u> may have forgotten it, but <u>I</u> haven't. You have, as usual, pushed it underground, in favour of that sickly niceness you know so well how to project. And don't maintain that Labour won the election on the strength of its policies: what was the real reason? The gullible public was persuaded, by such policies as were advanced, that they, the Labourites, were entitled to anything they wanted – it was theirs by right, they had only to demand it. This, apparently, is democracy: demand and supply. And Labour supplies it. Amongst its bountifulness is the promise that, if the working man does as little as possible, he will be rewarded with the maximum; this has become the unspoken but inalienable law. Complicit in this contract are politicians, intellectuals, and social activists alike, plus, of course, the working- man himself. The Social Contract has it that man was put on earth to enjoy as much as possible without actually earning it – an idea inherited from Marxism – and that as a consequence the government was in place to provide free handouts to all you lazy buggers who have been determined since birth to do nothing. Why bother, after all? The Welfare State is here to cater for all our needs; if you get V.D., pop along to the local hospital and they will cut your chopper off free of charge; the idea of paying for it doesn't arise, because the working man is not expected to earn enough to make a contribution to anything but the beer he drinks – and he can usually find the money for that. The working man – we'll call him Joe – is not expected to earn much because he is not qualified; and he is not qualified because, as we have seen, he has been determined since birth to do nothing. The Welfare State <u>is</u> necessary. Having decided to do nothing to justify his existence, Joe is encouraged in his idleness by the generosity of the State, which relieves him of the necessity to work, and, at the same time, of any guilt he may happen to feel. Marx, and a few psychiatrists, tell us that it is wrong to feel guilty because it makes us unhappy, and as a result those whom we have harmed go unsuccoured and un- apologised to; which I suppose doesn't matter if Joe carries on oblivious to it. The Welfare State is thus designed for the happiness of all of us – particularly those at the bottom, like Joe. What the State doesn't realize is that Joe isn't entitled, by any natural or spiritual law – or any law whatever – to anything but the socks he stands up in. Somehow Marx and a few psychiatrists have convinced the State that, contrary to expectation, God no longer exists; what he did before he died is either unspecified or hastily forgotten, and I, personally, am unaware of any reason why God would have taken it upon himself to die in the first place. However, I do know that when God <u>was</u> alive, he whispered in the ear of those few intelligent enough to listen that <u>man is entitled to nothing.</u> And ever since, in the minds of the intelligent few, this fundamental fact has been preserved. But in the minds of the unintelligentia, where nothing much but straw resides, a World Plan has been drawn up; and under this Plan, the idea has somehow come about that God, when he was alive, <u>was a liar;</u> that he deliberately told us the untruth that man was never destined to have any rights whatever – contrary to the frenzied protestations of every civil rights worker. But God foresaw – presumably before his death – that a plague of civil rights workers would infest the earth, bringing about the destruction of all those natural, and divine, laws that were designed to guide us through evolution. Because of this, evolution has come to an end; we are stuck in an impasse between truth and untruth, the truth being that Individuality is the Law, and the untruth being that the world is designed <u>for the common man.</u> The common man will never become an individual; he is too stupid, he is too indolent; he will never bestir himself. He nevertheless demands that everything should come to him; and the Welfare State, of course, gives it to him.

Society was intended for the individual; it thrives on individuality, which contributes to the welfare of the whole by energy and intelligence, and, by self-motivation and self-betterment, fulfils the purpose of evolution. But behold! What do we have? We have a society ruled by the Plan, which dictates that no-one need do anything, that certainly no-one should be forced to do anything (not even if the fate of the universe depended on it) and that if the world, in view of this, is to continue, then God, from beyond the grave, presumably, is to provide – or alternatively, Gordon Brown.

The Plan, of course, is designed by man for the express benefit of that lazy bugger, Joe, of whom, unfortunately, there are so many that they make up the bulk of society, and when these troglodytes work up the energy to vote, is it any wonder that the Conservatives never get in? So trammelled are we by Joe and his mates, that the whole social and governmental system is weighed down by a bureaucracy employed entirely for their ends; far from being a society run by individuals, it is answerable fundamentally to a population of useless layabouts. And if you doubt this, take a look at the vociferous majority before you; the common man, accounting for three-quarters of the population, is so mentally inferior – and no amount of education would have altered that – that he has neither the wits nor the determination, nor even any intention, of dragging himself out of his miserable condition. This, if he had the will, he could do, like the other quarter who have actually exerted themselves. No, he has not been 'kept down'; his own fecklessness has kept him from rising. How is it that the rest of the citizenry has bettered itself? But rather than put himself to any trouble, like going to a technical college or undertaking an apprenticeship, he prefers to seek the approval of his mates, who, under no circumstances, would exert themselves, and who, under this determination, impose their will on the weaker members of the fraternity. So, weak-willed and under the thumb of his associates, our hero proceeds through life like a piece of flotsam adrift on the tide of fate – blaming everyone else for his plight, as he has been instructed to do by all those authorities from Marx downwards – particularly the Nanny State, which was set up specifically to confirm and perpetuate this belief. And ever since, Civil Rights and Social Justice have ruled the roost – woe betide anyone who gets in their way.

A Final Note

Two further illusions advance themselves. First, the disgraceful illusion that there is any poverty in this country – apart from the disgraceful poverty of the pensioners. What poverty is there, may I ask? Everybody has a television, a roof over his head, a square meal at least once a day; no-one goes around bare-foot, all the kids have pocket-money (a thing which I never had) and the plea that some people are 'homeless, and sleeping on the streets' is answered by the fact that no-one except a tramp needs to be without a bed; anyone without a bed and a 'roof over his head' is so by choice; let there be no doubt about that. The council, in its weakness, provides for all: hostels (which are never full), bed-and- breakfasts, bed-sitters, homes for down-and-outs. Money is no problem, being doled out by the D.S.S. Go to Russia and China to see poverty. 'Poverty is relative', you say: richness is also relative.

Second, the David Davies farce. I used to think that Davies was intelligent, but he has let himself down by promoting the idea that civil liberties should take precedence over national security; 'our freedom is being eroded by further and further laws', he complains. Well let me complain that if we did not have the maximum security measures, we wouldn't have any freedom in the first place, because Al-Qaeda would be bombing us into oblivion. And if the police are asking for more time to question their suspects, obviously they need more time – otherwise they wouldn't be asking for it; and how does David Cameron know how long it takes to question a suspect? The Nanny State has been caught with its bloomers down again.

I do not mean to impugn the positive side of Tony Blair – he has done a lot of good for the country, and his concern for public welfare is genuine – but this is a veneer; as with all human beings, his positive exterior is belied by a devilish interior. Outwardly his career is marked by a distinct success – a success which disguises a very, very ambitious and ruthless determination. For years, Blair's positive exterior fooled me into thinking that he was 'a very nice chap'; but at the same time I had the nagging feeling that all was not right; such a pleasant impression could not possibly tally with his past, nor with the reality which I knew very well lay hidden behind that mask; persona and character have always been subject to the chaotic relationship of Jekyll and Hyde – which affects all of us.

Tony Blair is so concerned with projecting his image of niceness, that he would never believe the actual truth. He looks very nice, doesn't he? – smiling and smirking with complacency as he downs yet another Tory adversary with that calculated perversion of the man's argument: under that schoolboy's grin lies the insatiable heart of unquenched Ego.

In modern civilization, the surface show of positivity – and I admit it is positive – is actually a disastrous illusion; under it lies the Primordial Beast, untamed since the beginning of so-called 'evolution'; in fact, life, or the progress towards civilization, has never achieved its intended goal, humanity having failed miserably to embrace its obligations to itself. The positivity we exhibit is the only evidence of civilization, the underlying ninety-nine per cent of reality being repressed, partly out of necessity but largely because of our downright ineptitude – a fecklessness common to all men.

This is the reality behind all human beings: downright hatred, absolute egotism, murderous intent, and total savagery. In the depths of the unconscious, we find our true selves – the instinctive, treacherous, constant belligerence between each other and against ourselves; the oh-so-nice exterior, the socially acceptable persona, is a complete blind, set up to disguise these very facts. Unfortunately, evolution demands it, from a society which does, when all is said and done, have to defend itself-against itself.

It has to be faced.

Which is the greater reality: the one per-cent of niceness, affecting us all, or the ninety-nine per-cent of nastiness, also affecting us all? To which do we address ourselves, with a view to self-correction?

The Result of Humanity's Fundamental Schizophrenia

The fundamental reason for man's failure to accept Christ – and he is here today – is the condition of schizophrenia lying hidden within all human nature, from psychiatrists upwards. The schizophrenic condition has affected man ever since the dawn of consciousness, <u>consisting, basically, of the schism between consciousness and unconsciousness.</u> The very thing which was sent into the world to cure the disastrous effects of unconsciousness, has resulted in a universal illness based on that very fact; consciousness is the direct opposite of unconsciousness, and they do, and always have done, fight like cat and dog. God could not have produced a more destructive state of affairs; unfortunately, even God is not absolutely blessed with foresight, and if he were, the whole purpose of Creation would be nullified. The universe, with man at its centre, was invented as the mirror in which God reflects himself; that mirror is consciousness – God's consciousness of himself. Man was put on earth, as God's partner, for the precise purpose of facilitating God's mirror; the two of them together reflect each other.

Creation is an ongoing thing; it consists of evolution – it evolves. It evolves on the basis that one day man is going to take over from God; that is God's wish; He is grooming him for it. To that end, man must become conscious – to assume responsibility for himself. Civilization, therefore is man's consciousness, designed specifically to counter Nature's unconsciousness, which, though it may be essentially innocent, has yet a destructive side. Good and evil arise here, on the construction of civilization over Nature; consciousness and unconsciousness have been at each other's throats since Moses threw down the tablets of stone.

<u>Everyone does in fact recognize Christ, this being the very reason for his crucifixion.</u>

We have God against Man. It is a distressing and incredible fact that almost every member of the human race resents God's superiority; <u>this is the reason for rejecting him, in the person of his Son, and finally for crucifying him.</u> Man's pride, and even woman's to a lesser extent, will not let him acknowledge that anyone at all is his superior; fortunately, in most cases, this does not reach consciousness – when it does it results in certifiable schizophrenia – but we are left, nevertheless, with the schizophrenic illness – no less pathological. And because the basic fact about schizophrenia, whether normal or certifiable, is that the subject believes he is God – and this is almost invariably the case – there is obviously no room for manoeuvre between man's illusion and God's reality. <u>Man's unconsciousness is what leads him to kill the truth, or he who represents the truth;</u> it obscures the conscious perception of the truth, by withdrawing all recognition of the facts before him. We are not conscious of the ego within us and consequently it rules our lives, causing us to go against our better nature.

Unconsciously, everybody considers himself to be a hero; though he may consciously be unaware of it, it is this very conviction that prevents him regarding anyone else as being in an advantageous position; consequently fights, wars and all inter-personal strife are precipitated by the unconscious, raging beast of jealousy, by the urge to assert one's own right to equality, or superiority, in the face of all reason. Because men are not all equal, and Christ in particular is superior, the truth can not be admitted – man would be shown up for what he is: the sinner, the egotist, the coward; therefore he will not submit himself to the proffered salvation. The messenger of God is thus rejected on the grounds of his own creatures' self- aggrandizement. Can you give me any other reason why psychiatry and humanity in general condemn Truth on sight, whenever it appears? They cannot see Truth, being blinded by their all- consuming conceit.

(Addendum to every psychiatrist who has known me)

The Collective Unconscious, or One Mind, knows

everything, indelibly and undeniably. Therefore, when I walked through that door, you knew at once who I was – through the unconscious grapevine. Christ's presence is unmistakable, even though unconsciously perceived.

Knowledge of all is immediately present in every one of us; it so happens that, since birth, we have been accustomed to denying it. And what makes us deny it is Ego: 'Curse every messenger from God, for he makes us look small – in our own eyes'.

Misdiagnosis

I must reluctantly complain that you have not answered the most important and pressing question in my last letter, to wit, 'Do you believe that I am a schizophrenic?' The fact that Wittgenstein was diagnosed as such is neither here nor there, and I do not take kindly to being coupled with him. It seems you have ignored my very detailed explanation of how I came to be in psychiatric hands. I did not, of course, explain exactly why I was diagnosed in the first place; this is a matter, or an occurrence, which has never received acknowledgement from any subsequent doctor. You may not believe my account of what happened, because in common with most psychiatrists you probably assume that I am subject to imagination if not actually a liar – particularly in view of the fact that I have been a hospital inmate on many occasions, these occasions having come about through nothing to do with mental illness. I won't go into details, but my hospital incarcerations were entirely due to my original diagnosis, which was used as an excuse by many family doctors – that is to say GP's – when I approached them with a purely physical ailment[*]. It seems that having once been branded as a schizophrenic, one is presumed to be suffering from this very illness every time one comes down with the flu. Once in the hands of psychiatry, one finds it impossible to disentangle oneself.

As to the diagnosis itself, it came about in the following way. Having been admitted to hospital for what was admittedly a psycho- somatic disorder – though certainly not a serious mental illness – I was arraigned before a panel of doctors, who proceeded to bombard me with a series of inane and irrelevant questions, some of which were actually offensive. I was so incensed by their assumption that I was an incapable idiot that, when they finally asked me, 'Do you hear voices?' I shouted in reply, 'Yes!' This

---

[*] See Apendix

was quite contrary to what was actually the case; I have never heard voices in my life. It is a fact about myself that, when confronted by something, or someone, offensive, I take the most direct and counter-offensive attitude that could possibly be calculated to confound my adversary; so, therefore, when asked such an obviously insulting question, I immediately responded by declaring the exact opposite of the truth. This may seem illogical; but you must realize that I was not in a logical mood. In fact I only hurt myself; still less did I realize the consequences.

Obviously, when telling a psychiatrist that you hear voices, you are letting yourself in for a lifetime of harassment – which is exactly what has happened to me. Ever since that trivial event, I have been harried from pillar to post, in and out of hospital like a yo-yo; the slightest protest on my part has been received with dire suspicion and has usually met with downright suppression; the more vociferous my protest – and I can be very vociferous – the more severe the measures taken against it. Eventually, I became so demoralized that I actually accepted it, realizing that this was going to be my life until I died. Being a mental-patient is bad enough, but being drugged against one's will, and thereby losing all control over one's thoughts and actions, has to be experienced to be believed. The desperation I was reduced to truly merits my identification as 'The Prisoner'.

My past life, endured, no less, as the actual 'Man In The Iron Mask', has literally been a quest for my true identity, which has been hidden from me for something like sixty years. The undoubted truth that I did, actually, hide my identity from myself in no way alters the extreme suffering that I have always known – suffering which, I may say, it is impossible for the human being to even imagine. Not only has this suffering been mental, but it has also been, to an even greater extent, inflicted on me physically – entirely by myself. I have no one else to blame.

I suffer from exhaustion – extreme exhaustion – and though I am not touting for sympathy – a thing alien to my nature – this fact should be known; only through the most intense travail has Parsifal finally realized the goal of his life-long journey: not just his own identity but also the prize of consciousness. Parsifal's consciousness has been won in the Battle For Life, particularly in the development of a universal compassion; compassion itself, born necessarily of extreme experience, has brought about our hero's Awakening – resulting in 'The Theory Of Everything'; this exposition is nevertheless subordinate to Parsifal's mission to save the world by Example.

As we know, Wagner identified Parsifal with Christ – a truth shouting itself to us for the last two thousand years. I do not expect you to believe that I am He; I am after all suspected of insanity, and unfortunately human beings will always take the way of least resistance. Therefore it seems likely that my case is hopeless.

I may well die unrecognized; the rejection of its own saviour is the way of all flesh. The very people whom I have come to serve are the ones most likely to condemn me. My Crucifixion – gone of course unnoticed – is actually over; my Resurrection, while being perfectly evident, is yet to be announced. The last fifty years of my life have been passed in the Gulag, where, despite the attempts of life to extinguish me, my capacity for survival has preserved me; the Living-Death, which I not only represent but also actually am, is the Cross. The Christian Cross represents the tension between all opposites, including those of Life and Death. Impaled, as he is, on this Cross, Christ endures the schism between existence, or Life, and non-existence, or Death: spread-eagled between the two he is the Living-Death – holding out the promise to mankind of Eternal Life.

The concept of Eternal Life has moved on during the last two thousand years; it no longer represents the continued existence of life after the event of death. I come to proclaim the <u>existence</u> of life <u>within</u> death, the two together furnishing the Eternal Present, where past meets future, and future meets past. Thus, time and space – and consequently you – are stood on their head; no longer will man think in terms of 'life after death', or 'past and future', but in the very much more modern terms of 'here and now'. Everything will be revealed by Christ as the personification of Heaven Upon Earth, or <u>consciousness</u> – the former domain of heaven – <u>within unconsciousness</u> – the former domain of earth. Again, the two together result in the Supra-Conscious – the repository of past and future, life and death, and time and space.

The Eternal Now, or the 'here and now', will be realized here on earth, and no longer will there be any need to fear death. I promise it; I <u>am</u> it.

This illness consisted of uncontrollable vomiting due to the extreme anxiety resulting from my identity crisis. I have at last cured it, over the last five years, as a direct consequence of 'writing my way out of it'; in other words, I have become myself, thus resolving the crippling identity crisis.

The vomiting sickness was regarded as a manifestation of schizophrenia, which, I suppose, is inevitable if you make the assumption in the first place that I am a schizophrenic. The original diagnosis resulted directly from my exasperated outburst, and my apparent declaration that I 'heard voices' was something I regarded as so obviously untrue that no-one could possibly believe it – which is precisely why I said it.

ADDRESSED TO MY PUBLISHER

On the assumption that you are either an atheist or an agnostic – and I would guess the latter as you seem to be intelligent – it is my intention to convince you of my identity by means of evidence backed up by logic – which if it doesn't result in recognition, may at least persuade you to have your knackers looked at – some good may come of it.

Fifty Years in the Gulag: The Crucifixion

I am the Slayer, sent to kill man's ego. To that end, it is my very love for humanity that I have to overcome; hence, my Crucifixion.

The one basic desire in my life, the desire that pursues me throughout the day, is simply to lie down and die. This overwhelming craving has been the reality of my existence every day for the last fifty years – every day, all day, without relent.

Everything I attempt to do is vitiated by exhaustion; the slightest movement is an effort. Indeed I am a living-death.

You will be totally unaware, as is everyone else in the entire world, of your prophet's very real suffering. I will not go into detail, but suffice it to say that my everyday experience is so unimaginably awful that the only relief I have is in virtuoso swearing. I know every word in the book, and then some; my vocabulary is so extensive, and correspondingly colourful, that the air is constantly blue. I specialize in the worst, and deliberately most obscene, terminology that has ever been dredged up; everything I do and every object I come across, calls forth this response – from having a shit to tying up my shoe. Even the slightest movement is accompanied by a curse – such a struggle do I have to even exist: I am not alive.

My language is legendary, and my capacity for invention would surprise the most hardened trooper. I am willing to bet there have not been many prophets, sent from God, who resorted to such violent expressions; I am the most unholy of holy-men.

It is, indeed, the <u>only</u> relief I have, and without this outlet I would never have been able to continue. I am not asking for sympathy; that is the last thing I want, but I do have a right to make the world aware of the reality of their prophet's lifelong crucifixion – after all, it is for them.

Among my many identities, I occupy the character of Frankenstein, literally embodying man's attempt to create a living being, only, unlike the legend, I, or Frankenstein, <u>am creating myself</u>. I am the first self-made human – that is to say, the first actual individual – in history. Everything in my body, let alone my mentality, has been resurrected from lifeless tissue, I as a person having been dead for fifty years. My body has been totally dysfunctional all of that time, <u>the only animation having come from sheer will; I am will.</u> I represent will, I bring will.

Walk, I cannot; speak, I cannot; it is as much as I can do to lift my little finger. Struggling to perambulate, I make my way down the street like a strangulated chicken, attracting every jibe that you can throw at me; and being Frankenstein, I will one day turn on you. Make no mistake about that.

My chief concern is to re-create the universe in consciousness;

that is to say, I intend to raise <u>man</u> to a consciousness <u>of</u> the universe, the universe itself being supremely conscious. As part of my sojourn here on earth, I undertook a prolonged term of imprisonment in the Gulag, not least out of sympathy for those poor people in Russia. Admittedly <u>I</u> did not suffer from lack of food, but while their exhaustion <u>was</u> caused by lack of food, my exhaustion already existed; while most of them eventually died, I already was dead. In both cases unrelenting work was imposed on us; and in my instance it was a matter of flogging a dead horse. This regime resulted in my exhaustion being re-doubled; to that extent, at least, I was alive. But throughout the day I was hardly able to stand up, let alone walk, and from the moment I started in the morning it was my fervent wish that the end of the day was already there; in fact I had to pray for the strength to carry on from moment to moment, and this is actually what enabled me to endure it (apart from the copious swearing) because I learnt to live by taking one moment at a time. You might ask why I didn't retire into a lunatic asylum (free board and lodging). That answers itself.

<u>Incredible as it may seem, this is no exaggeration,</u> and my ability to survive it can only be accounted for by the fact that I am not an ordinary human being; if I had been, I would have gone under at the first step. You may wonder why all this went unnoticed by my colleagues, and indeed, if they were reading this now they would react with incredulity and fury – fury because they simply would not accept that anyone, particularly myself, could be capable of such an exceptional feat; and they will undoubtedly condemn me as a liar, especially as they did not observe anything unusual at all; but this was due partly to my very unusual powers of endurance, partly to the fact that I had no-one but myself to appeal to, and partly due to an innate ability to mask my pain. All this, however, was subordinate to what was perhaps my most valuable asset – my unfailing good humour. Even in the darkest hour, when I am practically on my knees, I come up with some quip that not only saves <u>me</u> but keeps the workplace going at the same time (it is not for nothing that Parsifal is known as 'The Holy Fool'). No-one suspected the truth for a moment, but I honestly think that the main reason was simply that man himself is born blind to his own Maker.

If I could not have got some humour out of the situation, it is likely I would have gone under. Through a combination of joking and swearing, I have enabled myself to survive – and for no other reason. I have never received any aid from the medical profession – indeed their contribution has been downright obstructive – especially where psychiatrists are concerned. I did nevertheless have one or two jobs which were comparatively light, but even then I had to pace myself by working in short bursts; I would put all my effort into a few minutes' work, and then hope for some time to recover. This did not always happen, due to the requirements of the job, in which case I simply had to soldier on. My ability to disguise my true condition was partly induced by the need to fool the authorities into accepting me – rather, that is, than sacking me. At the end of the day I would stagger out, cross-eyed with exhaustion, with the sole intention of collapsing as soon as possible. This has been my unremitting fate for practically the whole of my life; and again I say, this is literally true, and although I fully expect my former workmates to deny it – with venom – I do, in justice to myself, and of course in support of my mission, need to force this unwelcome fact onto the consciousness of the public. I have not come for nothing, and my life's story is essential history.

I reiterate, also, that under no circumstances would I ask for sympathy; I have never received any – expressly not from my mother, who might have been expected to notice something – and I do not expect to. This whole fifty years of crucifixion was brought on myself quite deliberately, and not only was it willingly undertaken, but I would not, for anything in the world, have missed it. It has been a truly epic battle, and it has left me strong.

(I often swear at myself – and bitterly – when I have otherwise failed to persuade myself to move. I thus drive myself even when there is no physical possibility of movement – which there normally isn't. Again, I say, this is no exaggeration. It has been a triumph of will – the ultimate triumph).

I have to repeat that, on no account whatever, can I permit you to even suspect that I am mentally ill. The uncontrollable vomiting was the direct result of my identity crisis, and therefore cannot be considered a normal manifestation of illness: indeed it was actually pre-ordained, the purpose of which will become clear in the near future.

How would it be if the Lord of the Universe <u>were a fucking madman?</u>

I am not telling you all this for nothing; I am ringing your heart-strings for a purpose. It should never be forgotten, or even doubted, that Christ's crucifixion is <u>real</u>, and that this extreme of suffering is designed to demonstrate God's overwhelming love for his world. If this <u>is</u> doubted, the whole contract between God and his people becomes nullified.

And if you personally doubt anything I am saying, I will cut your fucking balls off.

I live in a perpetual state of Nirvana – that is to say, the Supra-Conscious. I am the Supra-Conscious; otherwise I would not be privy to a theory of everything. Nirvana does include, you may be surprised to know, the most extreme experiences of suffering: that is its justification. No man will ever experience the ultimate enlightenment without the obligation to take on the suffering of the world – why else do you think man is exhorted to become a Buddha? – of which there have been many. And it is for this reason that Christ is crucified every two thousand years – a reasonable interval, in my estimation.

Have you not asked yourself why I have come at this time? Two thousand years, almost to the day, have elapsed since Christ last trod the earth; at that time, a crossroads of history, the world was in ferment – a particularly appropriate condition for the reception of the saviour. Today, when the world is in a greater crisis than ever before, it is an even more appropriate time to receive this saviour. At the present crossroads of history, when the old world is giving way to the new, and when every opposite is at the other's throat, is it not likely that God would have dispatched his son to save the situation?

And if you doubt my authority, just remember I am doing this for you, Mark.

Here is a list of my purely peripheral afflictions (starting at the top):

Feverishness and dizziness, leading to imbalance

Dandruff

Baldness, due to illness

Devastating headaches

Hay fever (in summer) a major affliction

Facial rash (recently disappeared) actually 20 years ago

Blurred vision, double vision

Eyebrows descending into my eyes, causing extreme irritation and obscuring vision, and impossible to get rid of; eyelashes constantly become entangled, again obscuring vision

Missing teeth for lack of energy to clean them

Nose constantly blocked, obscuring breathing

Throat constantly blocked due to polyps, adding to inability to speak

Bad breath, due to the ferment in my stomach, caused by anxiety

An almost total inability to physically write, due to jerking, and other manifestations. My rather good handwriting is totally deceptive, due to extremely laborious and time-consuming measures to achieve it – including constant correction of every word, and almost every letter in that word, due to illegibility. Writing is literally torture, and takes an incredibly long time

A complete inability to speak, unless I use the utmost will to feign it

Flatulence

Diarrhoea (a story in itself)

An itching arse, and constant need to urinate; Itching arse disappeared a year ago.

Unco-ordinated feet and legs, due partly to the complete inability to walk unless I am unconscious of it (which is never) being further exacerbated by exhaustion. I defy anyone to walk consciously

This all causes extreme physical frustration, quite apart from my totally incapacitating exhaustion, and long ago resulted in a complete, bloody mess – in a word, Frankenstein.

The above is all produced by the imposition of consciousness over every one of my instincts; but it is, or was, entirely necessary – and intended from the beginning. Instinct and consciousness are perhaps the most basic opposites, and for that reason were chosen to form the battle-ground on which my life was founded.

As they say: 'Physician, heal thyself'

———————

In regard to my misdiagnosis, I would point out that it rested solely on the incident I have described, and no succeeding doctor has even bothered to examine me, relying entirely on the original notes; but even on such scant evidence they have refused to acknowledge my frequent pleas that I am not mad, despite my repeated provision of proof that the diagnosis was mistaken. Their attitude stems not just from pig-headed stupidity, but more fundamentally from personal and professional ego, which I will not go into any further here. Thieves hang together.

None of these doctors ever saw me for more than five minutes every six months – the normal period; is that a basis for diagnosis? In contrast to the diagnosis by <u>one</u> doctor, on which the case rests, there have been no less than <u>five psychoanalysts</u> who have proclaimed that not only was there no evidence whatever of mental illness but also that <u>I was the up-and-coming prophet of the age.</u>[*] I defy you to disagree with them; and if <u>they</u> could see it, why couldn't the other bloody fools? These psychoanalysts, independently, and at the very first interview, knew right away who I was. It was that obvious.

---

[*] Two of these psychoanalysts – one of whom was actually a psychologist – did not actually hail me as 'the prophet', but merely as 'a genius' and not 'mentally ill'.

Whether you believe this or not, I obviously cannot persuade you, but it is a relevant fact that these psychoanalysts saw me solidly, every day, for four years – for an hour at a time. Who are the more likely to have known me? In addition, as you know, hard-headed psychologists don't go around declaring people prophets without a bloody good reason.

Two of these analysts appeared, in actual fact, twenty years after I was misdiagnosed, thus adding force to my claim, and though they immediately came up with the same conclusions as the other three, this was never made known to the psychiatrists who were actually in charge of me. I had gone to these analysts independently, for a second opinion, unknown to my tormentors; and for reasons which I myself find hard to credit, or understand, I did not repeat these findings, thinking that the analysts would have passed this on, but owing to the fact that my relations with them were unofficial, being unknown to the psychiatrists, and also because I never told them I was under medical supervision, this did not happen; and though I should obviously have been aware of their omission, I passed the rest of my life oblivious of it, and consequently was never able to understand why so many psychiatrists continued to believe I was insane. Sod's law. Nevertheless the two latter analysts impressed on me the necessity for giving up the drugs, which I could not do because I knew very well that they were the only thing, at that time, preventing my vomiting.

As you can see, my history is very complicated – and fraught. But I do have to tell you of another complication that will partly explain my acceptance of my supposed illness. Owing to my bouts of uncontrollable vomiting – the original reason for my being in hospital – I was put on drugs, and though they actually succeeded in suppressing this effect, I was totally unaware that they were also designed to treat schizophrenia – thanks to the misdiagnosis. For years I was oblivious of this, though from time to time I did suspect it. Throughout these years, also, I was unaware that I <u>had</u> been misdiagnosed, the precipitating incident having failed to alert me to this fact – which just shows how naive I was. I only realized the true state of affairs when, at the age of fifty, I was suddenly informed by a medical friend of mine that my drugs were really designed for this much more serious illness. I nearly had ten heart attacks: for the whole of my life I had not only been regarded as a madman, but I had also been subjected to drugs quite unnecessarily and probably with a distinctly harmful effect. The effects of schizophrenic drugs are largely unknown, apart from the fact that they appear to suppress the illness, and are not at all understood, and it is highly likely, as is believed in some quarters, that they would have a very undesirable result in other unpredictable ways. There is indeed strong evidence for this, and I myself have observed many schizophrenic patients gradually declining into a state of vegetation as a direct result. So, yes, I was less than delighted to receive this news.

It is only in comparatively recent years that I have at last attempted to disentangle myself from this web, largely because I incomprehensibly continued to believe I was a schizophrenic, due precisely to my friend's revelation; after all, if so many doctors over so many years had believed that, who was I to disagree? It only later dawned on me that this whole disastrous saga originated forty years ago with my exasperated outburst. I am not so far gone as not to know that I have never in my life exhibited any traits of schizophrenia whatsoever – despite what demoralization and self-doubt have served to convince me of.

My terms in hospital, I may add, were indescribably awful, locked up as I was with hordes of lunatics, drugged, against my will, into near oblivion, and with no hope of escape until I was finally released up to nine months later; in the meantime I was deprived of even the most basic privacy, and utterly unable to write, which was my only solace and my sole reason for living – the withdrawal of which left me literally as a walking corpse. I was even unable to think – the only distinction between a human being and an animal – and I would sit in a corner for hours, day after day, waiting solely for the event of my release. This, of course, was the final evidence the doctors needed to conclude that I was subject to 'paranoid fantasies' – what else could I be doing? The fact that someone could be so miserable that he simply sat huddled in a corner did not occur to them.

I did manage to force myself occasionally to do a bit of reading, but the word is indeed 'force', since I had an almighty struggle to take anything in even for a few minutes, and the book was shortly discarded. This was regarded, though, as an improvement in my behaviour, and was largely responsible for getting me released.

The 'House Of The Dead' wasn't in it.

If this hasn't rung your heart, it fucking well should have. I do not want your sympathy, but I do want to know that this has registered; <u>so do not omit it in your reply</u>.

This, after all, is my greatest reality – the reason for which I have come, thereby bestowing on me <u>the right to know</u>. Do not forget me.

WHO WOULD BE A PROPHET?

Perhaps the most unendurable part of my crucifixion – and make no mistake – that is what it was – was the unremitting ridicule that I faced every day; from walking down the street to the humiliation of hearing myself attempting to speak in an acceptable manner, when I was obviously failing to do so, I was subjected to the torments which only Frankenstein was destined to endure. <u>Again, literally true; and I defy anyone to contradict it.</u>

Frankenstein's body – and in the legend he apparently lacked a mind – has been subject to almost endless physical afflictions, chief of which have been the inability to walk and the imposition of a virtually total lack of co-ordination; in other words as I have mentioned several times, he has been unable to move. Quite apart from his mental afflictions – one of which is the withdrawal of the power of speech – this lack of movement is experienced purely physically, but he is nevertheless able to imitate movement <u>by sheer will,</u> as I have said, and no other being is able to do that. Frankenstein's whole life is governed by an act; a desperate attempt to present some semblance of animation; this results, usually, in a failure to be convincing, and he is thus the butt of everyone's jokes, due to the ridiculous figure he cuts. This, again, whether you care to admit it or not, is the absolute truth; Frankenstein is being crucified daily on the cross of ridicule.

You will be unaware of this, not having lived in London while I was there; it is perfectly obvious that you did not, because if you had you would undoubtedly have heard of me – and witnessed Frankenstein in action. Everyone in London, over sixty or thereabouts, will testify to this – except those of a similar mental background to yours, who have been so preoccupied with their own egoic affairs that they have simply remained ignorant of my existence – that being all the more incredible considering the resounding impact that my original discovery produced. I was known all over the world; Buddhist monks from various parts of Asia visited me, though some remained suspicious and resentful, resentment appearing to have been the chief reason why certain people did not accept me, especially in the case of the Muslims generally, who seem to grudge the fact that the representatives of any other religion have a right to exist. This collective egotism is largely responsible for the aggressive excesses committed in the name of Islam in recent times. I have no hesitation in condemning what appears to be a natural extremism at the root of the Asian psyche. In contrast to Islam, however, the religions of Hinduism and Buddhism were set up expressly to counter this disastrous tendency, whereas there is no evidence at all of any attempt on the part of the Muslim religion to regulate the play of opposites. Islam comes from the desert, where both nature and the indigenous peoples reflect the harsh reality of absolute dichotomy. However, in many parts of Asia, there are Muslims who have adopted a temperate and harmonious way of life that contrasts directly with the character of their religion. They are not ruled by the priesthood.

I make no apology for this digression.

As well as being visited by monks, I was sought out by ordinary people from many countries, some of whom actually came to work with me in order to enjoy my company. You may, as I fully expect, call me a liar; but I would ask, if I had not in fact been famous, how would these dear people, in those far off countries, have come to hear of me? I cannot, of course, prove that they actually came, so I might just as well retire for good into the mute hulk of Frankenstein from which I lately came.

My main effort has been to live within death, and the fact that this has not always been successful is responsible for my failure to convince. There is, nevertheless, a wealth of life within Frankenstein, prevented from expression by the inadequacies of his body. But this life is constantly struggling to get out, which is responsible for Christ's devastating conflict: to be or not to be; a conflict which has in itself reduced Christ to the shattered wreck you see now; and make no mistake, either, this is the reality of myself – Anthony Wakefield Hill, Jesus Christ, Frankenstein. Whichever of these you choose to call me, they all refer to the being who you presently witness in such a desperate plight; and it is desperate – it has been desperate for the last relentless fifty years – a further reality which needs to be recognized, otherwise the legends of Christ and Frankenstein will never find their predestined awakening in the figure of Anthony Wakefield Hill.

Anthony Wakefield Hill himself awaits resurrection, parading about in the meantime like the ghost of death warmed up. <u>When Christ awakes, the whole world will tremble</u> – and believe me, this will be the case; I intend to make it so. So watch out, all sinners – the Wrath of God is coming.

What people are laughing at is the figure I present, which results from the titanic struggle between life and death, and though it may appear hilarious, there is a shattered heart within the clown.

The crucifixion of Christ has 'passed on' over the intervening two thousand years; it has developed from a purely physical experience into what is now, in contemporary times, an essentially psychological experience. Christ was originally crucified on a wooden cross; I am being crucified on a cross of rejection and ridicule, due to the blindness, or unconsciousness, of man. That is why it is so important that you personally should be in no doubt whatever that I am not mad; otherwise our relationship can not possibly continue.

Two thousand years ago, the psyche of the common man was contained almost entirely within the body – if it existed at all. To exist, the psyche needs to be conscious: 'I think, therefore I am'. The most obvious characteristic of man at that time was his total unconsciousness; therefore Christ came to him in bodily form, the only form which man was capable of recognizing and the only basis upon which his mentality – not psyche – was founded; a body is capable of seeing only a body. The body can indeed contain the mentality, and in primitive man the mentality is so slight that it cannot peer over the parapet of its encompassing darkness. It is only in comparatively modern times that evolution has brought us to the brink of a conscious psyche; for the first time, man is beginning to think for himself, and, to inaugurate the forthcoming era of conscious psychology, Christ has come again, this time to be crucified in the guise of an hallucinating lunatic. And psychiatry has done its best to produce this outcome; sacrificed on the cross of perverted psychology, the man intended to be our saviour languishes unrecognized.

The Grail

I have just been listening to the prelude to Wagner's 'Lohengrin'; it features the appearance of the Holy Grail, rising gradually from out of the mists, the music reaching an almighty climax just as the Grail becomes most prominent; issuing a golden, resplendent light, sent especially to save man by the very power of its symbolism, it eventually recedes, back into the blue, as mysteriously as it arose.

The Holy Grail has been transformed into my Sphere, which retains the essential characteristics. Wagner foreshadowed it, I have brought it. From now on it will appear in the consciousness of man, not having previously emerged from the unconscious depths until Wagner became aware of it. It contains the power to cure all suffering, whether physical or mental – as we shall see in my next book.

The Holy Grail itself, originally in the form of a goblet, contains the blood of Christ, spilt in sacrifice for the world, for the very purpose of saving it. It symbolizes the Universal Libido, in all its aspects, which, as well as representing Christ's blood, holds the power to heal thus conferred on it. It also possesses the power to transform, which endows the Sphere itself with the same properties, and as I have elsewhere indicated, libido is the actual transforming agent behind the universal process of conversion – even to the nuclear conversion of energy. Among the many guises into which libido transforms <u>itself,</u> are the cosmic laws designed to facilitate the healing powers emanating from the heart of the universe, these laws being dependent on the intelligence of humankind for their implementation.

The spherical form of this new symbol represents wholeness, integration and the totality of reality, upon the contemplation of which rests the power to heal. <u>In the form of the goblet, the Grail</u>

represented the unconscious tradition of belief, for two thousand years; but this, admittedly effective, inspiration remained without the power to awake, and now finds itself overtaken by the demand for proof and reason in modern times, which we will see realized in the very modern form of the Sphere. The Sphere specifically emits the heavenly light of Consciousness, sent to awaken man, and to guide him in his further journey through evolution – evolution being nothing but the furtherance of consciousness, and having nothing to do with Darwin's obsession with monkeys. The one is the purpose, the other is the unfortunately blind process, out of which Christ has come to drag us.

(I should point out that the significance of the Sphere as a healing instrument is being fully described in my present book, 'The Revolutionising of Medical Procedure' – though I hasten to add that this substitution for traditional medicine is most certainly not 'faith healing' or anything irrational; it is in fact based entirely on reason and logic in the most practical application possible).

This will, I hope, give you a faint idea of my experiences – and I mean faint, their full extent being quite inconceivable to man. I have been to the ends of the earth and back, and let me tell you that God's capacity for suffering, in the service of his creation, is infinite, and never to be forgotten. Think not that he is up there sunning it with his angels (which, by the way, do exist).

That this extreme suffering – this whole extraordinary episode – has passed entirely unnoticed is due partly to my own prodigious self- control, but mainly to the deliberate refusal of humankind to acknowledge its own saviour – despite the overwhelming evidence. The signs were there to be read, and the only one with an excuse for not reading them was myself.

What the world has been witnessing, entirely unknown to itself, for the last fifty years, is my Crucifixion. It is now witnessing my Resurrection, which has been received by psychiatry as yet further evidence of my undoubted insanity; and my drugs have been re- doubled on the strength of it. However, my incriminating vitality and passion, because they are so extreme, could not in reality be attributed to anyone but a god – and I make no bones about that. This vitality has only lately been released, thus giving rise to the suspicion that my illness is worsening. The occasion of my Resurrection was first proclaimed by 'The Knowledge Of Everything' which could not be recognized as the work of anyone but a prophet. Could any human actually be in possession of the knowledge of everything?

Strangely enough, the one thing I have never been accused of, until very recently, is the claim that I am Christ, or some other prophet. <u>The reason is that I never have claimed it.</u> Over all the years that I have been reputed to be the prophet, <u>I am the one person who has denied it</u>. And that is why I am ill. I wish it to be known categorically, and without the slightest doubt, that far from claiming that I am in any way exceptional, I did in fact break with the psychoanalysts who saved me, on this very point; because they trumpeted the fact that I was Christ, and treated me for four years on this basis, I, as a reasonable and modest human being, could not bring myself to accept it; and so I broke with them. Does that say I am a schizophrenic?

Sad as this was, it was pre-ordained, because I had to go underground – another story.

Although I say I have never claimed to be Christ, I have in fact claimed it on two occasions – and of course to my Stepmother – once at the beginning of my career, and, recently, right at the end.

On about the first occasion I was in hospital, and for reasons which I have not time to go into now, I claimed, under the utmost embarrassment to myself and with the greatest unwillingness, that I was the prophet. I was forced to do this by circumstances which I do not expect you to understand at this point, since I have not time to describe them. But let it be understood that I only did this under extreme duress, and I have never uttered a word of it since. It resulted in my being detained in hospital for months, until the original analysts came to my rescue again and convinced the authorities that, despite what I had said, I was in fact sane; the authorities then, apparently, accepted along with many other people at that time, that I was the prophet.

I do not know what has been recorded in my notes: whether I have been accused of claiming I am Christ, or simply that I have 'heard voices'; either of these could have resulted in my diagnosis, because the doctor who actually diagnosed me, on a later spell in hospital, may well have remembered my original claim, and despite the analysts' good work have reverted to the former belief that I was mad; this would be confirmed, of course, by my apparent statement that I heard voices – a very complicated business, and I wouldn't be surprised if you didn't believe a word.

It is only in the last two years, after sixty-odd years of denying my own identity, that I have finally been forced to acknowledge it, one reason being that the only alternative is to commit suicide. And I cannot do that, because, thank God, I realize the world depends on me.

Do not think that I have chosen self-belief as an easier option than suicide; I am no stranger to suicide, having been on the brink of it every day of my life, the only thing preventing me being the knowledge that my loved ones would suffer even more than myself as a result – or so I thought. This, though, was the sole reason; suicide would have been a welcome relief, and those who <u>have</u> committed suicide can count themselves lucky to have escaped the continuing experiences that have fallen to my lot.

You may thank your lucky stars that I have not done this.

I don't think that even now I would know who I was if it hadn't been for the timely intervention of those five psychoanalysts; it is certain that I would not otherwise have the courage to believe it: after all, how many people can call themselves the Son of God?

It has been borne in upon me lately that the overriding reason for my failure to accept myself is my reluctance to don the mantle of the Avenger, or the Scourge of God, which I am and which I have to be. My fundamental experience, since coming to earth, has been an overwhelming sympathy for mankind – my people – and as a result of my acute awareness of their problems and suffering I have felt the greatest and most unconditional love for them; that is why I have come. But along with my love, there is the equal obligation to take the world to task – in fact to accuse them of wrong doing and generally give them hell. Only by doing this will I be able to change them; it is a necessary preliminary to my teaching. I will in fact have to wield the big stick; it is absolutely no good pussy-footing about, as, unfortunately, so many people do. Humans need authority and stern handling, otherwise nothing can be accomplished. Therefore I will have to shout and swear at them (at which I am a past-master). But as you can understand, I am approaching this with the greatest unwillingness – so unwillingly, in fact, <u>that I would prefer to sacrifice my own life in order to avoid it</u> which is precisely what I have done. That is crucifixion.

<u>This is the reality of Christ.</u>

And if you don't believe it, you can shove it up your fucking arse.

I have poured my blood out for this world, and I do not expect it to be thrown back in my face. I want commitment, and I am going to get it: that means an uncompromising declaration that you believe in me. You have all the facts; it would take someone with the mentality of a psychiatrist – in other words, a Barbary ape – to ignore them.

Epilogue

Life is a battle; and the battle
Is the prize.

Christ and Schizophrenia

INTRODUCTION

I have suffered seriously from nausea, resulting in uncontrollable vomiting, since I was twenty-five, when I was first put on drugs, having come to the notice of psychiatry. Although, to all appearances, this condition was out of control, it was, as I have said, not subject to the normal criteria of illness. It actually turns out to have been subject to Christ's own will, and in fact, over the last five years, he has succeeded in curing it by will. That is to say, he deliberately set out to cure it, and has done so; this has been accomplished basically by my decision to 'write my way out of it' – a very salutary process, and to be recommended. Without going into details, let me just say that I intentionally took myself in hand, and 'persuaded' myself that vomiting was no longer necessary; the whole point being that, originally, it was necessary – as a disguise for my underground journey, which the illness initiated, and sustained throughout. <u>Without it no one would have thought I was ill</u> – and my mission as Parsifal would never have come about. The whole thing was designed and controlled by myself, deliberately set up for the purpose of being finally ended by the application of my own will – a procedure which I intend to establish as the basis for my future teaching and healing. Will, of course, is necessarily accompanied by logic and reasoning. But if it had not been for my self-subjection to a devastating illness, the underground journey would never have occurred, primarily because there would have been no cover for it – but also, of course, because the illness itself was designed to be the inspiration for my awakening – or enlightenment, in the tradition of the Parsifal myth.

I could have stopped this illness in a trice, at any moment, <u>but 1 had to hide myself from myself,</u> and the drugs were applied in direct support of this necessity – though not, of course, within the consciousness of the psychiatrists, who were an unwitting instrument. The drugs, furthermore, served to maintain <u>my own unconsciousness,</u> without which Parsifal's journey would not have been possible, since he, or I, would have been supremely conscious right from the start, which would have rendered the whole of my mission redundant. The whole of my life, up to the present time, has been necessarily unconscious, leading, so painfully and so gradually, to my ultimate triumph as a conscious being – not, indeed, for my own sake, but for that of humanity; witness the Imitato Christi, the whole idea of which is projected by the peregrinations of Parsifal's psyche – an undertaking required of every human being.

As for the analysis of schizophrenia itself, the most obvious thing to strike the observer is the fact that, whereas a normal person <u>is two people in one</u>, the inevitable schism being contained, a schizophrenic <u>is simply two people</u>, with no connection between. This is what the drug attempts to cure, or would attempt if it were designed to. In so far as Christ could be described as a schizophrenic – and there are undeniable similarities between his affliction and the mental illness – this would only hold true if Christ himself were two unrelated people; but as this is demonstrably, and unmistakably, untrue, the question does not arise. The idea that Jesus' crucifixion is in any way a mental illness, is too preposterous to be considered. Suffer, he did – and mightily – but this was designed right from the start.

The Cross itself is a symbol which could give rise to the notion that it represented schizophrenia (if anyone were intelligent enough to think so) – if regarded superficially – but the Cross also represents the healing function, in other words the Third Element, or the all- containing whole which synthesizes the pathological gap. It is on this basis that I propose to treat schizophrenia. Nevertheless, it could be said that Christianity is responsible for the widespread occurrence of this devastating illness (again, if you were intelligent enough) through the very schism it undoubtedly symbolizes. But then, was not this schism always present in the world, awaiting the advent of Christianity, and the Cross, to heal it?

A Drug Designed For Schizophrenia

About forty-five years ago, a drug called L.S.D. was introduced for the treatment of schizophrenia. It was also known as the 'truth drug', and was aptly named, being applied for the specific purpose of revealing to the patient the nature and cause of his illness. That drugs do not actually contain the images they are intended to inspire, but only have the power to induce them, is something so obvious that it has never occurred to anyone. The images arising in a person's mind have always been there, waiting to be brought out by some benign, or malign, drug; but as the effects on the patient are, predictably, so extreme, the authorities have withdrawn the use of the drug. A pity, because it is the only effective treatment for schizophrenia, <u>and its extreme effects are not due to the drug itself, but entirely due to the traumatic nature of the illness.</u> So, again, human rights have done man a disservice, and no schizophrenic would thank you for it. We have been deprived of a salvation sent by Nature's own solicitude.

The truth drug is designed to present to the patient a <u>picture of himself, in the very images arising from his own mind</u>: it is not hard to see that the truth already exists in the patient's unconsciousness, <u>and he knows that</u>. The extreme effects are produced solely by the patient's insane resistance to the truth; insanity itself is simply a denial of reality – a denial which is deliberate on the part of the patient, <u>being put in place by will, and therefore removable by will.</u> No patient is without hope, as long as he is also guided by the wise ministrations of the psychiatrist. He has to be reduced to the rock- bottom reality of his own nature; this is the true location of hell. The mental patient has to be confronted with himself, and he will discover that, like all other human beings, he is a craven coward. If you, the reader, do not recognize this as yourself, I strongly recommend that you get in touch with a therapist.

L.S.D. is the most merciful, and most effective, instrument in the armoury of the psychiatrist, having been withdrawn in the mistaken and weak-kneed assumption that everyone is as pusillanimous as the withdrawing authorities themselves, who in reality should be on the sick-bed. The truth drug succeeds on the same basis as my shock-treatment, both being designed to rescue the patient from his self-imposed imprisonment in darkness, by the God-sent means of consciousness, induced, unavoidably, by strong measures. I will therefore lobby for the reinstatement of L.S.D.

In my case, the application of L.S.D. had very salutary, though sometimes horrific, effects. I was enabled to see, as was intended, the nature of my illness – the nature, but not the cause. The cause of my illness remained a mystery to me until recently, not least because, as the psychiatrist said, the cause would probably not become evident until twenty years later, this being normally the case, the assumption being that the patient would not until then understand why he had become ill, though obviously he would meanwhile be able to deal with it. Consciousness, apparently, does not dawn on us until we are forty.

I had, perhaps, fifteen doses of L.S.D., and the effects ranged from the hilarious to the most incredible suffering. Although these experiences obviously came from myself, I was not conscious of that at the time, but although the doctors thought I was too far gone under the drug to be aware of my surroundings, or conscious of anything at all, I was in fact completely conscious all the way through, being entirely aware of my surroundings and also of the fact that I was under drugs. However horrific, and extraordinary, my experiences were, I never succumbed to unconsciousness – _and that is precisely why I suffered so much_. Despite everything that has been thrown at me, over the whole of my life, I have never lost consciousness: I _am_ consciousness. Therefore no drug, except a mental one such as an anaesthetic, has been able to reduce me to the state desired by the doctors, and though I may have been physically incapacitated by tranquillizers and sedatives, which were designed to put me to sleep, this did not result in mental unconsciousness – I only wish it had. This fact, I am sure, will result in fury on the part of the doctors and nurses who were in charge of me – what impertinence! – and they will undoubtedly go out of their way to try and disprove it. How could he be so exceptional! Sorry, boys, I <u>am</u> exceptional.

My first dose of L.S.D. resulted in a brief episode where I was stuffed down the funnel of a tramp-steamer, churned around in the engines, and finally spewed out of the bilges into a sea of shit. This is, indeed, my life-story, and I recognized it, from the drug-experience, a few years later; my original wish as a child was that I should experience absolutely everything, good and bad, and that I should be thoroughly used up – even abused – by life itself. Otherwise there was no point in living; you must be a hostage to life. And so it has turned out to be; I have indeed experienced everything, being churned around in the engines of life, within the bowels of my very shabby vessel – I was, for forty years, a mangy kitchen-porter – and spewed out, much to my disgust, into the enveloping cess-pit of existence. Yes, I have seen the world <u>from the arse up. How do you think I know so much?</u>

However, I got more than I bargained for. Even before my prolonged battle with the sons of psychiatry, I was a white-haired veteran of a hundred existences; literally true, since, by the time I was twenty, I had experienced as many as that of a hundred men, and knowing that this will be received as a grossly exaggerated claim, let me try a little proof. When I was a boy of ten, my hair was bright red; when I reached the age of twenty, it had faded to almost white; almost, but not quite, because red hair never loses its colour until right at the end of a man's life, unlike other colours, which may deteriorate comparatively rapidly from black to grey to white; and as you all know, it is not uncommon to see a man with practically white hair at the age of thirty, which would not be attributed to any unusual circumstances. It is in fact a natural occurrence. But in my case, it was far from natural. Red hair, over the course of a man's life, may of course fade, reaching a state of near-whiteness at, say, the age of sixty, but, before that, it forebears to go grey, proceeding from its original brightness to <u>lesser shades</u> of brightness, and under natural conditions the colour would not noticeably change, until its owner had reached a very advanced age. Under conditions of illness, black hair may go grey, and it does not take a very serious affliction to cause it; how many men have you seen walking about, perfectly happily, with grey hair – completely unaffected by physical suffering?

(and do read this, you bastards)

The claim by my family that my hair took on its present colour by a natural process – and the complete denial that it had lost its colour by my twentieth year – may, by stretching the bounds of credulity, be attributed to their constant proximity to me; but surely this very proximity should have alerted them to my extreme condition? From which it would follow that the colour of my hair was most certainly not indicative of a normal state of affairs.

<u>I am not asking for your sympathy, you cunts.</u> But I do get angry when my own family denies, with the utmost venom, that I have suffered the tortures of the damned – both physical and mental. Indeed, I am the damned.

Though I subjected <u>myself</u> to physical torture, I expect my experience to be acknowledged, especially as it was undertaken on your behalf. Through it, I have learnt how to rescue you; so for that reason, honour it.

By the time I reached twenty, my physical experiences alone had reduced my hair almost to the colour of white, and it would actually have been white if its natural pigments had not persisted where the pigments of other colours are destined to fade. Do I make myself clear?

————————

Another interesting experience that I had under L.S.D. was neither hilarious nor horrific. It was just a Fact; a fact I observed when I was transported into outer space. I observed that existence was an illusion – the first time that I became aware of this singularity. I witnessed not only that nothing existed, but also that existence itself did not exist – not even the concept of it. You might ask, did I myself exist? <u>The only reality I had was as the observing power;</u> I, at least, could see that nothing existed, and I was left to infer that consciousness was the only possible form of existence; as long as you can see, therefore, <u>you,</u> exist. And that which you see only exists in your mind; that which you see, is seen, and thereby attains reality. So consciousness sees that which it is conscious of; hence the idea that existence is a mirror to God: <u>that existence is a mirror reflecting God's mind.</u> And therefore we conclude that existence only achieves reality in the mind of man when man realizes that nothing exists except mind.

This latter fact totally eludes science, which is stuck in the belief that nothing in fact exists except the physical universe: the exact opposite of the truth; and this illusion leads to the further illusion that God himself does not exist; the scientist cannot see God, therefore he concludes that there is no reason <u>to believe</u> he exists, whereas, because God is consciousness itself, the scientist cannot see what is to be seen, not being possessed of the most elementary consciousness.

It is a fairly common assumption among philosophers that 'existence is an illusion'; in fact it is not only an assumption, it is also an affectation: it is <u>clever</u> to say it, and fashionable. They cannot see it, and they cannot prove it.

In reporting this experience, afterwards, to the psychiatrist, I announced: 'I don't know what God is' – meaning that I did.

I now come to the most singular of my L.S.D. experiences – in fact the most appalling experience of my life. I was shown myself as I was – what I was actually suffering from – and at the same time, I experienced the suffering, which was my normal condition, <u>a million times more intensely than I had ever before been conscious of</u>. This you will immediately dismiss as 'not possible'. I am not a liar; I do not exaggerate – in fact, on this occasion I am understating the case. I am at the centre of the universe; I keep it going. I experience, at the centre of the universe, the collision, or tension, of opposites; this tension is what enables the universe to exist, and I support it, and suffer from it personally, all day and every day. Whether you believe this or not, it doesn't alter the facts. How do <u>you</u> know, anyway? Have you ever been to the centre of the universe? Have you any knowledge at all of metaphysics? – of what determines the construction and process of the universe? Unless you are equating yourself to Christ, you would have no idea what the universe consists of. I myself, quite apart from the testimonies of five distinguished psychoanalysts, have experienced and seen enough of the world, from the arse-end up, to know that I am not mad, and to interpret the revelations which are sent, via the truth-drug, to instruct us as to reality. <u>These pictures of oneself do not lie:</u> their truth is inescapable, and does not give rise to mistaken interpretation. <u>Indeed, if I had been a liar, and a paranoid fantasist, that would undoubtedly have been shown up by the drug.</u>

So, then, you may by now be receptive to my description of the experience. Without further ado, I am going to announce myself as Christ; <u>I</u> know I am not mad, even if you don't. Being Christ, it is not unlikely that I would suffer as Christ – and suffer, I certainly did. I was, in fact, strung on a wire; and though this wire did not actually exist, I have to use the description to convey my meaning; which was that I was the victim of the most refined torture ever devised by God. And the only justification that God has, is that he is me – his own son, in whose person he has come to earth. This schizophrenic condition is well known to followers of the Church, having been proclaimed ad-nauseam by the Bible and other means; the extraordinary thing is, nevertheless, that no-one has ever realized that it is actually schizophrenia. We are told, on the one hand, that Christ is the Son of God; on the other hand, we are told that God himself came to earth – to sort us out. Where no-one makes the connection, despite the blindingly obvious implication, is in the inescapable conclusion that Christ and God are one. And also, despite the whole Christian message to this effect, not one solitary human being has taken it on board – except, evidently, myself, who have been aware of it practically since birth. <u>The schizophrenic condition, therefore, rests not in God but in man.</u> God is conscious of his own dual nature; therefore he cannot possibly be schizophrenic, a condition which is defined by unconsciousness. But man is not only unconscious of God's condition, he is also unconscious of his own, which is basically pathological; there are vastly more schizophrenics walking around the streets than there are cooped up in hospital, unknown to themselves precisely because they are unconscious. <u>Schizophrenia is a condition affecting all of us. and there is no such thing as a normal man.</u> The only difference between the man in hospital and the man in the street, is that the latter has not been rumbled – and I intend to do that.

That is what I have been sent to do, <u>and it is the collision</u>

between this obligation and my love for humanity that has resulted in my crucifixion – which might well be considered schizophrenic. It is the condition of crucifixion that I experienced under the drug, and though it is bad enough in my normal waking life, it received an overwhelmingly increased effect on this occasion; no-one would believe the power of this drug – but then, it wasn't the drug at all, but my own revelation to myself, redoubled on two counts: first, the nature of the conflict itself, and second, the desire of someone somewhere to indicate to me that this was my situation, of which I was normally totally unconscious, apart from the very definite suffering. But the effect was redoubled by the ongoing conflict, which had the weight of the universe behind it, and also by the very attempt of someone to present me with the picture. The intention was thwarted by my own inability to grasp the situation, until a few years later, when it was explained to me by my angelic psychoanalysts. In this instance, the truth-drug was unsuccessful, because my need to disguise the truth from myself was stronger than my desire to save myself. This is the case right now. I have therefore to employ the truth-drug's revelations of forty-five years ago, which only now am I in a position to do. And thank God for that, the old buggar.

> I dreamt I was tickling my own Father's balls
> With a little sweet oil on a feather;
> Of a sudden I woke
> And I found it no joke –
> He was tanning my arse with a leather!

It's about time the old cunt realized his son has come of age.

The experience of crucifixion thus thrust in my face, was magnified to the extent that I was not conscious of anything else: I was crucifixion; there was nothing else in existence. My arms were outstretched in the crucified position, and I was so transfixed on the wire of tension, between my two arms, that I could not move in any direction; I could not escape the paralyzing and excruciating pain – all I could do was to hurl myself around in circles, from one pole of tension to the other, in a frantic attempt to obtain some relief – which I was utterly unable to find. I was within an ace of going irretrievably mad, and any ordinary being would have succumbed at once. It would in fact have furnished relief if I had gone mad, <u>but I was denied even this possibility by my own consciousness – the need to retain my sanity at all costs:</u> I must have realized dimly that the fate of the world depended on it.

This condition lasted – and, incredibly, this is true – for the best part of twenty-four hours – for the full twenty-four hours if you count the initial experiences. In the morning, I was issued with the drug, and I remained in a side-room until the afternoon, during which time I underwent such a severe trauma that I would not have believed it possible that it could be followed by anything worse – which it was. The initial trauma, I do not recall with such clarity, since it was superseded by the second, but I do recall beyond doubt that, inspired by the drug, I was lying on the floor of a prison – indefinitely. It is important to realize that this prison represented my life, or my psyche, <u>which itself had subjected me to imprisonment for, as far as I could tell, an indefinite period.</u> To that extent, the 'image' represented the truth, and it is a fact that I have spent the whole of my life since the age of ten in a physical and mental prison – imposed by myself. So what I was experiencing was an extreme of suffering within the walls of my own prison. I am afraid I cannot describe the physical and mental experience itself; that is something I cannot do even today, when this same experience is continuing. Suffice it to say that, even without the drug, it has always been unendurable – yet I have endured it, because I have no choice. And indeed it <u>has</u> lasted indefinitely.

The thing I remember most vividly, while lying on the floor in extremis, was my decision not to accept any drug designed to relieve me, under any circumstances whatever; <u>I knew that, if I did so, I would be finished. However bad I was, I had to endure it because consciousness supersedes all.</u> And so it has been throughout my life; I have never found the slightest relief for my suffering, and even if it had been offered, I would not have taken it.

The one thing I will say about this experience, and the one

immediately following it, was that they were both expressive of the same thing: Christ's Limbo. Limbo is a term often used to describe a condition in between two events; an interval where nothing happens. But in Christ's case, something most certainly did happen; although he was in a state of limbo, <u>in other words, a state of suspension between opposites, where nothing is supposed to happen, this suspension was fused with the extreme tension between those opposites. Hence. Christ was just one thing: tension: the tension between every opposite in the universe.</u> This is an unenviable condition, as you can readily understand, but it is quite beyond the human's ability to imagine what it was actually like – and what it still is like. Fortunately, in my normal waking state, the underlying condition does not penetrate, though, believe me, it is quite bad enough as a surface event.

This experience of limbo found its worst manifestation, however, in the further infliction of a sense of timelessness – the absence of a sense of time – which produced in one an impression of permanence, or a perpetual present; there was no past and no future, just an ever-present torture, with no hope of relief or even the hope that it would end: why should it, if it were perpetual? As far as I could see, I was there indefinitely, with no consciousness other than of what was happening to me. Nevertheless, I was from time to time aware that there was a nurse sitting it the room, not all the time but just occasionally. This nurse was there for a specific reason: <u>to refuse me any drugs which might relieve me,</u> and I did ask him twice for such relief. He remained stonily silent. No, you are not right in thinking this was my imagination, nor in thinking that, 'of course, the nurse wouldn't have subjected you to unnecessary suffering'; but that is just what he was there for. Before you dismiss this as fantasy, let me inform you of psychiatric procedure at that time. It was not an uncommon practice, in the case of an intractable psychosis, to subject the patient to extreme and deliberate trauma, in the belief that his illness involved the paranoid conviction that he was a hero. We know, of course, that this is invariably true of schizophrenic patients; so you can see the logic of it. Reduce the poor fellow to such a state of suffering that he screams, preferably in tears, for relief; and on being refused relief, he will be even further induced to beg on his hands and knees. Thus, the patient is brought face to face with his own cowardice – the cause of his illness.

I have witnessed this procedure many times, though by now it may have been discontinued, and it has been practiced on myself also many times – without result, I may add. To whatever extremes those psychiatrists reduced me, they did not succeed in breaking me – if they had, my suffering would have been relieved, instead of continuing beyond belief. The effects of the drug did not wear off for twenty-four hours – I was evidently given a good dose, which was probably boosted – and until it began to subside the next morning, I was in a constant and unrelieved state of suffering, so extreme that it could not possibly be described. I dare say that the psychiatrists, if they had had any inkling of it, might have put me out, but they remained aloof in the conviction that I must be shown up for what I was.

In this state of limbo, one is not conscious of anything but the suffering itself, so intense is it that it displaces everything else in the mind; the victim is not even conscious that there is such a thing as existence, his own existence consisting entirely of blinding pain – that, and nothing else. <u>The sense of time is gone, and replaced by eternity, and the present, simultaneously, so that one is only conscious, if of anything at all, of a present annihilation that at the same time goes on forever: the Perpetual Present.</u>

The state of limbo is thus the crucifixion of the universe, in which Christ is the representative figure. This is your saviour's reality; don't say I never did anything for you.

The Perpetual Present might be considered to be a positive and happy event, having been presented by myself ('Life And Death', from 'The Knowledge Of Everything') as the experience of Nirvana in its ultimate stages, and as the message of both Christianity and Buddhism when taken together. But it also entails a commitment on the part of the adept to undergo the suffering of his fellow humans – in the fashion of Christ if not the Buddha. But in Christ's case, this was taken a stage further-indeed, several stages further; he was in fact crucified. And crucifixion means taking on the weight of the universe in all its aspects; as I have described at length elsewhere, the universe consists of Mind – the collective Mind – meaning that every one of us is contained within this Mind. Our mind, whether that of the individual or the collective, consists, very basically, of the juxtaposition of opposites; and these opposites, under normal conditions, act in harmony. But owing to man's distinct susceptibility, the opposites are more often than not at loggerheads.

The opposites being at loggerheads, then, <u>the whole world is in conflagration.</u> Brother fights brother, whole nations are tearing each other apart, and on the home front we are assailed by the collision of spirit and flesh, truth and untruth, and good and evil in general. All a fine bloody mess, which Christ has come to clear up.

<u>By presenting man with a picture of himself, Christ intends to convey to him his infamy across the board, but more particularly, the means by which he can cure himself. And the picture that Christ presents is projected quintessentially by his own crucifixion. The Idiot that you see decimated on his cross, is none other than yourself.</u>

By observing Christ on his cross, man can learn what is wrong with himself, and how to put it right – if he is intelligent enough to read the signs presented for this purpose – and also honest enough. And do not be in any doubt of the severity of Christ's suffering on your behalf; he is undertaking it partly out of choice, but also inadvertently because of the schism within himself: the collision between his love for you and the need to chastise you. This is a situation which Christ finds it impossible to resolve: it is, in fact, his Crucifixion. Having been sent to earth to flay the life out of man, Christ finds it impossible to do so. The wrath of God which sent him has been assuaged by the intervention of the son against his father. But the task remains.

But right at the end of his crucifixion, when Christ finally dies to the physical world, he awakes to the Ultimate Consciousness, and becomes the Father, from whom he parted on his fateful journey and to whom he has now returned. The Son of God is indeed the Father, but only when he realizes this will his Crucifixion be ended: consciousness returns to consciousness, consciousness returns to itself. Thus the journey is ended – and, who knows, maybe all that suffering was worth it?

May I apply to Dr G, late of Garlands Hospital, to vouch for my sanity – then, as now?

APPENDIX

I have decided to add a further experience that I had in hospital, not unconnected with the foregoing – in fact, <u>directly</u> connected with it. This experience lasted even longer than that under L.S.D., though the drug administered was merely a sedative, or whatever you call it, designed to induce sleep. I will not bore you with the less horrific aspects of this time, which were at first largely physical, but they alone caused me the severest trauma; however, as they <u>were</u> basically physical, I will not recount them, except that one of them consisted of severe convulsions, which were very painful, and lasted through several interminable nights, though receding in the mornings when the drug wore off. This, as I now realize, was a side- effect, but it went entirely unnoticed by the nurses, who were too busy farting. On this occasion, too, I could only escape the pain by writhing from one position to another; though this was my intention, it did not actually relieve the pain, but merely enabled me to discover an alternative position from which to contemplate it. You may consider my capacity for endurance incredible; it is. My failure to notify the unwatchful nurses, was due to my belief that the whole thing was intended, and that therefore I would receive no sympathy, and I have never been in the habit of complaining anyway, a fact which has obscured my life-long suffering from the eyes of those who should have guessed it. When the nurses weren't farting they were asleep, or in their office talking. Whether or not my tortures continued the following day, when the drugs were re- applied, I do not remember, since night and day were blurred into one. My condition must eventually have been noticed, because, as far as I recall, it did finally recede – but this may have been because my body got used to the drugs – even drugs becoming fed up sometimes.

This marathon endurance test lasted weeks, and possibly for about two months, during most of which time I was forcibly detained in bed, <u>on the supposition that I was asleep. But in fact, during the whole of this unbelievably lone episode, I remained awake, being vouchsafed hardly a minute's unconsciousness.</u> The doctors will not believe this, since the drug was designed to induce sleep, and psychiatric drugs don't fail, do they? Despite these ministrations, I lay in bed perfectly aware of what was going on around me – day and night. There was actually more going on at night than during the day, since in daylight hours, most of the affected patients were asleep and the others were out on the town. At night, however, things became more active, from the administration of drugs to farting competitions among the nurses; the nurses had been told to fart as loudly as possible for my benefit, though how I was expected to hear them while I was asleep, I don't know. However, I wasn't asleep, and they were very entertaining. The charge-nurse's 'specials', delivered at great frequency, were the only light relief I had during my long ordeal – for which I am eternally grateful.

You may wonder why I dwell on farting; and I am not going to tell you, except that there has been a tradition in this country, ever since I came to fame, to regale me with 'nonsense'. Those among you under sixty-five, or who have been particularly unconscious for the last forty-five years, will not be aware of this. Though I myself have never been able to discover the reason for it, this practice has been constant throughout my adult life, but has met with furious denial, whenever I have mentioned it, from all psychiatrists under sixty-five, who are not in a position to know. So unless they assume that Christ himself is a pathological liar, I don't understand <u>this</u>, either.

The unrelieved state of consciousness to which I was unintentionally subjected, continued unabated, due, I have to admit, to my chronic need to retain my sanity – or the need to remain conscious in a desperate bid to preserve my thinking-life. This was under dire threat by the imposition of drugs, which, being designed to destroy consciousness itself, automatically destroyed the thinking process also. <u>And I mean destroy</u>. The doctors could not have done me a greater disservice: in trying to treat me for madness, they in fact imposed a regime which very nearly produced that madness; if I had not been mad before, I most certainly would have become so. Dr D, who appeared to be quite friendly towards me, was actually the chief architect of my distress, unwitting though it may have been. The train of thought on which I had been engaged for many years was submerged by the drug, and I don't think that, even today, it has re-emerged. Because I realized that this vital knowledge was slipping away from me – probably never to be recovered – I struggled like hell to keep myself conscious – and I succeeded, over a period of weeks if not months. I could not allow myself to sleep, except fitfully, because once that chain of thought had been broken, it was impossible to pick it up again; the underlying continuity was lost for good. The psychiatrists were informed of this by my uncle, who visited me in hospital, but even his good offices failed to persuade them to abandon their diabolical technique: once again, do not be fooled by the innocent face of psychiatry, which is all the more evil for its lack of awareness; evil is often worked most strongly in institutions set up to prevent it, and there is no excuse for being unconscious of the evil within oneself. <u>Evil is unconsciousness</u> and what could be more evil than the unconscious attempt of man to suppress his own saviour? – For this is what it amounted to. Dove and all the others were aware of my former identification as the prophet – hence his friendliness – but even though they were unaware of the reason for my diagnosis as a schizophrenic, they assumed, simply from my notes, that I was such. They did not attempt to submit me to analysis. Judged on my behaviour, I gave them no reason to condemn me; but Dove was not disposed to accept anyone as a prophet, therefore anyone who had such a reputation was automatically mad. In the absence of a reason for my diagnosis, his conviction that I was mad was a pure assumption: is assumption a basis for keeping a man in hospital for nine months? – without any behavioural evidence to support it?

Thus, Christ's Limbo was confirmed and perpetuated by the ignorance and blindness of psychiatrists who are paid to know better; they had the evidence before them; the same evidence that had led three hard-headed psychoanalysts before them to conclude that I was not only particularly sane but that I was also the finest brain in the universe – evidence that was so bloody obvious that all three of them accepted it on very first acquaintance. <u>They saw who I was immediately.</u> It was so unmistakable to them, that I am asking you, Dove, 'How come a cunt like you failed utterly to recognize me after I had been, for months, stripped naked in your own back- yard?'

And don't give me the line that you were treating me for vomiting. I wasn't put in hospital for vomiting, and I didn't vomit while I was there – except on one brief occasion when I was treated immediately and successfully by pills. Even if it had been decided to treat me for vomiting – which I didn't ask you to do – there was no excuse for keeping me in hospital for a further six months – unless your concern for me was so great that you decided to inflict even more torture on me. I could easily have been treated, if at all, as an outpatient. And the whole of my stay in that hospital consisted of the withdrawal of all my awareness that I was a human being – so far was I reduced. Your failure to realize this is incomprehensible in face of the evidence, which was blindingly obvious to those prepared to look. But then, psychiatry itself is distinguished by its abysmal lack of consciousness, the very quality it was put on earth to develop, in order to rescue its patients from the same darkness.

The person once reputed to be Christ – and I think even you were conscious of that – was treated, on the flimsy diagnosis of one doctor, as a grovelling lunatic – surely an abrupt transformation?

Lying in bed, therefore, in an interminable state of consciousness, <u>I was suspended from all life.</u> Incredible as it may seem, this is literally true, and though it is the permanent reality of Christ's own condemnation, it was neither relieved nor witnessed. The state of Limbo is exactly that: <u>a suspension in nothingness</u>; an area in which nothing happens: there is no evidence to the victim of any vestige of life within himself; he cannot consult himself. Being withdrawn from all daily activity, except for meals he couldn't eat, Christ was thrown back on his mental resources, which didn't exist thanks to the drugs. Though he was conscious, he was conscious only of his surroundings: he was not able to think – beyond the fact that he was <u>not</u> able to think; a reality which presented him with his own Crucifixion. Being unable to think, the only form of life available to Christ even under normal circumstances, he was reduced to the status of an animal – except that an animal does actually live. This state of suspension from all contact with life, except the bed-pan, was endured by Christ for at least a month, unremitting, and productive only of the consciousness of his plight – of the fact that he could do nothing about it.

The only life present in the Son of God is the capacity for mental reflection: that is his existence; reality consists, in fact, of thinking – the only reason for which we are put on earth – apart from eating and farting – and, of course, sleeping. But sleeping is precisely the thing we are required to overcome – by the application of consciousness <u>through</u> thinking. <u>So, if the capacity to do this is withdrawn from Christ, what is he left with? – Nothingness, limbo. Crucifixion.</u>

After a month of this, I was reduced to tears. That Christ should be reduced to tears is indeed an event. But let me say at once, that these tears were not produced by weakness; they were deliberately intended as a protest – not even as an appeal for help. I was not begging anyone to do anything, but by demonstrating to the doctors exactly what they were doing to me – and I could think of no other way convincing enough – I hoped to bring an end to this intransigently inflicted suffering. No, it was not weakness. And if you do not believe this, I can only put it down to your own ego, which is saying, 'I would break into tears, therefore I don't believe anyone else is strong enough not to'. Modesty and swank combined – a condition affecting most doctors and nurses, which would logically disqualify them from office. I intend to carry out a purge of the mental health system; all doctors exhibiting any signs of egotism will be required to undergo analysis designed to expurgate it. This is supposed to be the regular procedure, but in my experience it doesn't work. In Christ's analytical procedures, fisticuffs is employed, and is so effective that most would-be psychiatrists would shit themselves for fear of displaying any ego. That is what God has set me on earth to do – boxing-gloves and all.

However, the one person strong enough not to burst into

tears, unless he decides to do so, is Christ himself; do you think you can break the Son of God?

But, observing my tears, Dove came up to me in delight and said, 'I see you're actually crying!' – the implication being, of course, that I was, again, a coward; an imputation that has many times been disproved.

Moving, now, to the question of physical cowardice, which I shall treat briefly although it is a large subject, I was hauled up, one day, to be interviewed by a visiting doctor (who evidently had not undergone sufficient analysis). I told him that this enforced suspension from thought had resulted in the decimation of all my ideas and philosophies, and rendered it improbable that I would ever recover the knowledge that had been lost, or even the ability to continue my train of thought in the future. His ego did not require him to be interested. When I said that, as a consequence, I would be unable to carry on my philosophical and proselytizing work, which at that time was widely known, this unfeeling and conceited authority, because his ego had not allowed him to recognize my own celebrity, sneeringly replied, 'What work?' – in the sense that I could not possibly have any important work – being a lowly schizophrenic.

On receipt of this answer, I retired, gob smacked. But so furious was I that I returned to the attack, and as a last-ditch attempt at protest, I threw a jug through the glass door (Christ does not disapprove of violence – especially when it is the result of desperation – and I have been desperate many times). This monstrous demonstration of aggression was immediately followed, you will not be surprised to learn, by Dove's decision to subject me to an operation without an anaesthetic; the assumption being that, as I was undoubtedly a coward – this being proved by my having the impertinence to assert myself – I would collapse in tears, thus revealing it. They were disappointed. The operation was a minor one for the purpose of applying stitches to the wound I had incurred from the broken glass. But during the lengthy application of the needle, I failed to display any reaction whatever either physically or mentally. Throughout my life I have been accustomed to bearing pain without showing any sign of it – a thing required of any prophet who proposes to challenge humanity to do its worst. This sort of thing is all in the day's work, and I have endured far worse. I managed to counter the pain by exerting all my energy against it, plus a few choice oaths, which went unnoticed by the doctors, being under my breath.

The result of my prolonged physical extremity was that my sensitivity had increased fivefold by the time I was twenty. I have told you before that even at this early age, I had already lived a hundred men's lives, both physically and mentally. <u>Incredible though it may seem, this is no exaggeration, and was only possible in the body, and mind, of a being selected for his superhuman powers of endurance.</u> My experiences started at the early age of ten years, and rapidly became extreme. All this, even more incredibly, has never even been suspected by my own family, my masculinity, itself being superhuman, having enabled me to disguise my suffering from them. My masculinity has always been disguised in turn, by my superabundant femininity, and therefore was not apparent to my family – who will deny its very existence. I have no reason to be thankful to my family: 'A prophet is not without honour save in his own country' – and in his own family.

But despite this greatly exaggerated sensitivity, the strange thing is that my threshold of pain was actually withdrawn, to the extent that if I cut my finger, I would not feel anything for several seconds – but then, the pain would kick in five times more greatly than originally. No, Mr Doctor, this was – is – not due to 'shock'; Christ does not suffer from shock; the delayed reaction was caused by the nerve- receptors' inability to register extreme pain immediately – precisely because it was so severe; they were overloaded. 'Rubbish. Nobody could possibly experience pain to that extent'. But I can; not only was my sensitivity increased, but it became so <u>tenfold</u>; <u>my innate modesty caused me to understate the case</u> – with my sister in mind, since she, under no circumstances would accept the truth, being convinced that she alone is born to suffer – by dispensation of God? I am not an ordinary person, and even apart from my greatly increased sensitivity, caused by an exceptional capacity for suffering, I am able to feel with the delicacy of the whole universe behind me – 'Rubbish!' Whence comes this psychiatrist? – so dismissive is he.

With the whole universe behind me, my quotient of

femininity is particularly high, but because my quotient of masculinity is also particularly great, I am able to endure pain to an extraordinary degree. However, my sensitivity over perhaps the last twenty years has accumulated so much that I am no longer able to resist pain to the same extent; in fact I am now one thing: overwhelming sensitivity. This has come about not least because of the incredible quantity of life bursting at my door; the whole universe behind me is desperately trying to push its way out; and my body, instructed by my mind, prevents it. Bursting at the seams therefore, having strained against instinct all its life, the body has become a vessel of raw nerves – that, and nothing else. So sensitive am I that, ten years ago, when I had my nose 'packed' after an operation, I screamed the place down; I do not know just how painful this process is expected to be, but the presiding doctor announced at the beginning that he was not going to give me an anaesthetic; I do not know what his intentions were, and he didn't tell me, but he certainly got results. The pain was excruciating, and partly because my resistance had been reduced so much, <u>and partly because that area of the anatomy is not easy to exert resistance on,</u> the only way I could deal with the pain was to scream. This was my way of resisting it; most people scream because they are not putting up any resistance.

Despite the fact that I said the pain was excruciating, the whole experience could have been that of a psychological trauma; the fellow was ramming a substantial iron spike right up to the ultimate reaches of the nose, without any great delicacy, and he eventually reached the area closely adjacent to the eye. I felt that he was inexorably driving the spike further and further into a highly sensitive area, and would not stop until he had penetrated my eye, and then gone on into my brain. This was something that I simultaneously felt and anticipated; a psychological trauma consists of two things: the mental image and the physical experience, psychology, or the mind, being a combination of the mentality and the body (something I have proved before). If my 'imagination' had been restricted to the mental image, the experience would have been a mental trauma and not a psychological one; hence, what I <u>felt</u> was the physical experience, and what I <u>envisaged</u> was the mental image. Whether the pain was excruciating or not – and I am not at all sure there wasn't some physical basis for assuming that – the experience was absolutely horrific, and the screaming may have been directed against the horror.

The upshot is that any psychological experience is a combination of mental and physical factors, a conclusion that could have a major influence on future medical practice.

My physical experiences have resulted, as I was told by a knowledgeable dentist, who had inflicted severe torture on me, <u>in extreme tension within my bodily tissues which is the cause of my physical susceptibility.</u> Whether the tension itself arose physically or mentally, I don't know, but I am indebted to this thinking dentist for revealing the reason behind my inexplicable condition.

It could be that when that particularly thick iron spike was forced up my nose, it did not take any account of the narrowness of the nasal passage, and owing to the tension of my tissues this could conceivably have caused the pain I have been complaining of.

Recently, a woman dentist, despite her personal charm, committed double murder on me. Because the aesthetic had not been delivered adequately – a common occurrence – I received the maximum pain, but when dentists have a time-schedule, they are reluctant to be held up by the need for another aesthetic; and knowing this from life-long experience, I did not attempt to persuade her, God having invested me with a long-suffering regard for the demands on a dentist's time. So I was left with two choices: either to resort to blubbing like a child, which is one way of dealing with it, or to resist the pain by swearing like a trooper; you will remember that my experience of pain is intense. Neither of these options would have been necessary in the case of an ordinary person, whose experience of pain in the dentist's chair, or anywhere else, is not great, despite their belief that they have undergone severe suffering, and despite their invariable claim that, for some reason they can bear pain better than a weakling like myself – the unspoken belief. I am regarded as a weakling by all and sundry, owing to their egoic assumption – in the same style as that of a psychiatrist, when faced with the subliminal opportunity to assert his superiority, despite his analytical training. Why else become a psychiatrist?

The expletives I used, having decided to adopt the measure of swearing, ranged widely, from 'you fucking bitch! you whore!' to the more intellectually informed 'you daughter of Satan!' I was thus enabled to endure the onslaught.

The dentist was unaware of the lurid descriptions of herself issuing from my mind, and because my resistance was so effective, she never even knew the pain I was in – unless she observed my desperately clenched fists. Believe me, any pain inflicted on myself is felt with incredible intensity.

This was the result of the actual extraction, but she prefaced it by not giving me any aesthetic at all, prior to the injection, on the roof of my mouth, an area particularly receptive to pain when one's tissues are extraordinarily tense. The front of the gum does not suffer so much – in the case of the injection – because it can be anaesthetized, as a preliminary measure, by a swab. The process of injecting me on the roof of the mouth caused even more pain than the actual extraction, and I could only deal with it by means of an alternative variety of expletives.

This has been, in part, an account of Christ's crucifixion. It did take place on a cross – the cross of opposites – <u>particularly the tension between.</u> Christ himself <u>is</u> tension, sent to endure tension, and thereby to save the world. Think not that he enjoyed his visit.

Psychiatry and the Inability to Think

For the last forty years, I have been regarded as a schizophrenic, and, on that basis, drugged into a condition of mental obscurity; that is to say, my mental powers were overcome by sedation, so drastically reducing my ability to write. For this, and the complete misdiagnosis in the first place, I have to thank the ineptitude and downright malice of psychiatry, a corpus of personages dedicated to the overthrow of reason.

Psychiatry in general imposes the very madness it is designed to prevent, this madness issuing, in the first place, from the mentality of the psychiatrist himself, which is no less than schizophrenic, as I shall prove. From the issuing mentality, the proposed imposition of madness descends on the patient in the form of drugs and other ill- conceived methods of treatment. So little is known of the nature of mental illness that, still today, nineteenth-century procedures and diagnoses are retained.

Being inspired from the outset by the doctor's inadequately suppressed ego, the diagnostic process consists initially of faulty observation, this being reinforced by a lack of experience in even the elementary knowledge of human nature; so ignorant are these 'experts' that they do not even know the precipitating factors of schizophrenia, which have to be assessed prior to diagnosis. (I am of course concentrating on schizophrenia, the most besetting of illnesses, most others merely needing a minimum of observation and knowledge on the part of the 'consultant'). It is the fashion, today, to assert that schizophrenia 'does not consist of a split- mind', despite the obvious meaning of the word 'schizo', which is 'split', or 'schism'. Whoever coined the word originally evidently did so on correct observation, <u>for the whole human race suffers from this Schism. from psychiatrists to prime ministers</u>. We have a country, therefore, led by schizophrenics at the top, and doctored by schizophrenics at the bottom: not a situation to inspire confidence in the ordinary man, or patient, on the receiving end.

Proceeding from the faulty observation, the doctor will pronounce his verdict: 'This patient is mad because I say so'. No reason will be given, simply a description of the accompanying symptoms, which apparently are assumed to be the cause as well as being the symptoms themselves. The description 'schizophrenia' arises from the assumption that the mere description confers the diagnosis; which would be true if the illness and the diagnosis coincided, but, as we have seen, owing to the faulty observation, there is a certain split between reality and the desired conclusion; the doctor's ego interposes itself here, persuading him to consult his inadequate experience in the hope of establishing a relationship between cause and result. This is not always possible, because in between cause and result there is always a world of possibilities which renders any conclusion difficult and therefore dubious. Two and two do not always make four – in fact, usually they don't – so the unfortunate patient is, on the above basis, subjected to a regime of totally unsuitable drugs (which are not, anyway, designed to actually cure the illness) and a programme of the most peculiar, and irrelevant, 'social events', which are evidently intended to promote his 'mental development'; these events, far from promoting his welfare, usually result in a tendency to depression, in view of their dullness and total failure to engage his interest. If he is conscious enough, the patient will probably wander down to the pub, when the ward doors are unlocked, and relieve his depression in drink (he may be an alcoholic as well) or retreat to the lavatory and relieve his tensions there in solitary masturbation. These extra-curricular activities are all that is available to the inmates – apart from 'occupational therapy', which no-one wants to attend unless the therapist has an unusually short skirt on, thus showing her knickers. This is probably the most positive treatment on offer.

LETTER TO DR G AND THE BODY OF PSYCHIATRY

If I get any more cheek from psychiatry, I will take the bloody lot of you to court. Yes, that is a threat.

In this volume, psychiatry is in for the biggest exposure of its history, right from the bottom up; I reveal every abuse and misdiagnosis to which I have been subjected over the last forty years – the physical enforcement of drugs in particular, which has, until recently, decimated my ability to write or even to think. In face of that, is it any wonder that I am angry? – But that's just mental illness, isn't it?

As to the question, 'Do I believe I am Christ?' in point of fact, I have <u>never</u> believed I am Christ. That has always been my problem, and still is my problem. Even today, when I have conclusive proof that I am the Messiah, <u>I do not believe it</u>. That is why I am ill, this diagnosis proceeding from no less than five psychoanalysts; can you, who have seen me twice for fifteen minutes go against the verdicts of three people who saw me every day for four years? But of course you would go against them, simply because I am telling you. You are determined to believe, against all proof and reason, that no- one in history could possibly be Christ because Sigmund Freud said so. Unfortunately you are unable to follow even this simple logic.

By your own admission, you haven't bothered to read it anyway, have you? Some basis for diagnosis

The diagnosis you possess in my notes comes from the last G.P. I saw in London fifteen years ago, not from any psychiatrist. The last psychiatrist I saw was a lady, thirty years ago, who discharged me from psychiatric care, saying quite categorically that there was nothing wrong with me, apart from cowardice. So, therefore, if you want to find out the truth about me, you will probably have to look at <u>her</u> notes.

All this is logic, which you cannot follow. So I do not propose to waste my time with you any longer. I do not give two fucks whether you believe I am Christ or not – I am not out to impress anyone.

However, my defence rests on my exposé of you and your colleagues, so I shall continue.

Your ego is king-sized, which is why you will not acknowledge me. Believe me, I know – I am the Healer and I can smell an ego a mile off. The fact that this is being aired in public is something you can't do anything about, because it is not illegal to hold people up to ridicule, which is how I propose to treat your ego. You see, you psychiatrists are in the unenviable position of not knowing anything; your egos have prevented it; yet you still practice diagnosis on the basis of ignorance. The fact that you are usually right, doesn't mean you <u>are</u> right, but simply that you aren't actually wrong ('thinking', you see) which in turn means that there is a lot of room for manoeuvre between observation and diagnosis.

By this time, as usual, you will have given up reading, if you started in the first place – but how do you expect to understand me if you do not read me? As I told that dunderhead, Dr L, how do you propose to conduct an interview without reading my history? How can you possibly interpret my behaviour? My 'behaviour', by the way, is described by the one intelligent psychiatrist I have ever met, as 'eccentric', and nothing more; he even accepted my shouting at him as normal and understandably provoked – and not in the least 'threatening'. I am an extremely vital, passionate and forceful man, and can sometimes, to the weak and impressionable, appear 'frightening': can I help it if someone is a weak-kneed drip, like yourself and Moosa? Is it 'criminal'?

Between the original perception and the eventual diagnosis, <u>there is a world of infinite possibility,</u> in which anything could happen – and, in my case, did – and which therefore means that any simplistic conclusion is highly suspect. For this reason, any diagnosis, despite the fact that it may be correct, is most unreliable and has no genuine authority. Psychology boasts itself as being 'an inexact science', so is there no room for doubt as to its assessment of myself? Psychologists may be right in their assessment of most patients – despite themselves – but mine is a case of 'the rule proving the exception'.

The act of diagnosis goes straight from the observation to the conclusion without any acknowledgement of what lies between, which is the only place where there could be any truth, and without which, any assessment, though it may be right, is incompetent – blind, in fact. The doctor makes the <u>assumption</u> that he is correct without actually knowing; the fact that he <u>is</u> correct is in no way due to his perspicacity, but due solely to luck. Anything he observes is based on prior assumptions, which are based on previous assumptions, and on <u>ever more</u> previous assumptions... All medical experience, however profound it is (that is, mental medicine) is approximate, and cannot be, by medicine's own admission, taken as gospel truth. And in my case, can you dismiss my reluctant claim to be Christ – despite the abundant proof and testimonies – as undoubted evidence of madness? Is it not possible for Christ to come to earth? – especially in the guise of an Idiot?

All of man's perceptive and cognitive powers are derived from the delusion that he can see and think. In point of fact he can do neither; he is neither conscious nor capable of applied logic. Any correct diagnosis, therefore, is a complete fluke, being dependent on non-existent logic and the most dubious experience.

The fact that Jones is a depressive does not mean that the diagnosis is accurate but merely that Jones is a depressive. The doctor has not proved by diagnostic powers that the man is suffering from depression; he is assuming, merely because he has walked through the surgery door, that he is suffering from something. In that, he is undoubtedly right – a monkey could see that for himself – but the progression from noting that the man is obviously ill – snot is probably running from his nose – to determining that he suffers from depression is a step that actually should include many steps. The attending circumstances, such as snot, may or may not indicate the source of the man's illness, but from our doctor's inadequate experience – even though he has been in the business for years – the deliberation of such a task would at best be approximate and at worst downright misleading – leaving sundry gaps for doubt.

I am trying to gradually build up a picture of man's inability to think, and therefore of psychology's incompetence to pass judgment. Judgment based on the incapacity to think can not be sound, man's deficiency in this regard being indisputable, he having but lately arrived from the apes.

Prophet's are fierce, and my anger is caused by an offence, not to me, but to the Truth.

It is the Truth that is offended, and in defence of the Truth I am prepared to express myself forcefully. That is evidently 'mental illness'.

As far as 'threats' go, the only one under threat is myself: the threat of incapacitating drugs against a professional writer who needs to be in command of his wits, and who has never had the accusation of 'mental illness' against him proved in any shape or form. And if I dare to protest at all, I receive the further threat that my drugs will be increased – as they have been. The enforcement of drugs, or any treatment at all, in my case is totally illegal and not even justified. No-one has ever proved that I have written dirty, obscene, or otherwise filthy letters; nor has anyone proved that I have ever written a threatening letter. I have proved exactly the opposite in a letter to the Chief Constable of Lancashire, and this proof has been accepted. I intend to put this whole disgraceful series of events forward in the next issue of this journal. Freedom of speech permits me to do so, and you can't touch me – unless you propose to threaten the Rights of Man as well?

Now as to the latest 'threatening letter':

The following is the letter I sent my brother-in-law in response to a most flagrant insult. It was the immediate cause of my being forcibly detained in hospital, coupled with my temerity in leaving off the drugs which interfered with my mental capacities, and were a gross imposition in the first place – all this despite the fact that I was a 'voluntary patient' for thirty-five years.

> 'You expressed the utmost contempt for me. I do not take that from any Irish peasant.
>
> I am not a man to take an insult lying down; very soon you will feel the weight of my fist.
>
> I hit particularly hard, having been trained extensively in the boxing- rings of Sedbergh – a thing of which most people are unaware. It is my intention, therefore, to drive your nose right through the back of your insolent head. Doubt not my ability to do it. Even in this obviously frail body rests the capacity to deal out the most severe punishment: I am who I am; and that will be proved in the press in exactly three months' time. Any doubts you may have of my identity will be resolved.
>
> I do not accept any attempt at an apology; that could only be a further insult. I hereby terminate all association with my family – including that bitch of a wife of yours.

For this missive, I was branded a 'danger to society', and awarded
six weeks in hospital (enforced, though I still am a voluntary
patient) and put on an accelerated regime of drugs – also
enforced. Apparently, if I had hit my brother-in-law, as I refrained
from doing, I would not have been regarded as a danger to
society, because actually hitting someone is not 'a threat'.
Threatening letters are not allowed under any circumstances –
however innocuous, and even in answer to a dire insult; perhaps I
should sue my brother-in- law in court? – Or better still, kiss his
arse?

Because they couldn't think of a better excuse to drug me,
they thought up the idea that my vitality and 'talent to amuse'
were evidence of manic behaviour; I am in fact a natural
comedian, and if a talent to amuse is a psychiatric offence, you
might as well lock up every comedian in the business. Even I
didn't go at it all the time; I gave them plenty of respite. But this
makes no difference when you are confronted with a South
African bitch who is determined to do you for something. Apart
from my flashes of ill-temper, resulting from the provocative and
impertinent behaviour of the doctor herself, I evinced unusually
good humour – also regarded as manic – because, despite my
incarceration in hospital, I had managed to continue my 'self-
resurrection', i.e. my self-rescue from my own, life-long
suppression. This filled me with enthusiasm, a thing that is not
allowed.

Whether or not you regard me as Christ – and I don't care
either way – Christ himself can stand most things – even derision
– but the one thing he can't stand is contempt – contempt
springing from egotism. And so, whoever expresses this contempt
needs to have his egotism expunged, precisely because it is an
insult to Truth itself. So I take the most direct and most effective
measures against P—. I had no intention of hitting him, though I
could have done.

That letter was not an expression even of my ire: it was simply
the execution of my process of putting down ego wherever I

encounter it. Whether or not you consider I have the right to do so, that is what I do. Whether or not you believe me to be the Healer, nevertheless I heal; and as you know, egotism is our primary enemy.

You have to understand from the outset that, wherever I come from – whether from heaven or hell – I have charged within me – even against my will – the obligation to cure man of all his ills, expressly by means of physical aggression. Aggression against aggression; there is no other means of fighting it; the traditional method of moral persuasion – whispering sweet nothings in his ear – does nothing to persuade a man that he is not God. And it is the belief that he is God, or someone like him, that drives man to assert his superiority. This is what needs to be addressed.

Now, I had always been of the belief that P—, above all people, did not suffer from egotism. But I am afraid he does. All the time I have known him, he has had a barely-restrained contempt for me; he has hardly had the time of day for me, and, recently, perceiving in me an abrupt change of character, he would indeed speak to me, but only reluctantly. This underlying attitude – unconscious on his part – led directly to his insulting dismissal of my attempts at conversation. Although there may have been other factors, and though my family thought the whole affair was trivial, it does reveal a fundamental pathology (which my sister will never accept). It is actually the cause of P—'s illness, his alcoholism.

No-one has been able to cure his alcoholism (or anyone else's) because no-one has ever known the cause of it. Now he has the God-sent opportunity to cure himself; I do not cure people, I merely present them with the opportunity to cure themselves. I reduce them to the quivering wreck of absolute self-dismay which they must go through before they can rise up, the New Man: the eternal Phoenix rising again from the pyre of Destruction. This is my procedure, my reason for being on earth, wherever I may come from and whether you believe it or not.

The actual state of affairs within P—'s mind is the classic Schism between conscious and unconscious. This invariably produces a conflict between the unconscious truth and the conscious denial: the fact that I am afraid, and the refusal to admit it. All soldiers are susceptible to this syndrome: the very nature of their trade makes them assume they are invincible; it is inevitable; and this, the unconscious truth, is forcibly kept underground. P— has always known the truth – that is why he drinks: he cannot face it. This is the underlying fact of most mental illnesses; <u>the egoic unconscious in conflict with the conscious truth: a fundamentally paradoxical situation. For, while the unconscious actually holds the truth, despite itself, the conscious has the power to deliver it – if it can be extracted from the darkness obscuring it.</u>

Squash the ego forcibly, thus presenting the patient with the unwelcome truth – a picture of himself – and, depending on his moral fibre, <u>he can take his life in his hands and begin to love himself.</u> He has to accept the basic wretchedness of all human beings – the one thing we are constantly denying – and humbly realize his position before God; for God, in fact, is the only hero.

And so I have reduced P—'s ego; I have released his unconscious – if he will acknowledge it – and he is now in a position to go forward.

As to that insolent sister of mine, she has to learn the same thing; she, also, suffers from abominable ego, and because, under no circumstances will she admit it – being incapable of seeing it – she persists in the 'conscious' belief that she is the angel of mercy sent to cure everyone else (an occupation, actually, which I reserve to myself). This is the inescapable and obvious reality behind my sister's lifelong attitude and behaviour, both towards the world in general and myself in particular. <u>Everyone in my family knows who I am.</u> and it has always been their determination to deny it and to put me down: why else but ego? No-one can admit that this idiot in their midst is actually the only hero in the business.

This will draw the most vicious fury – how could this insolent booby possibly accuse us of such knavery? We are above it! E—'s image as Florence Nightingale, which she knows so well how to put forward – and which was probably instilled in her during her days at Lowther – has to confront the unconscious reality of the intransigent hellion who tramples on every truth in her path, and who, above all, <u>lies to herself.</u> 'Know thyself', is the injunction, and everyone on earth does their best to deny it. Civilization, or the social front which we present to the world, only accounts for one- per-cent of our psychological make-up, the other ninety-nine per- cent consisting of raging savagery. This fact is known to some representatives of the psychiatric body but, unfortunately, not to most of them, despite its obvious presence in their everyday dealings with their patients: murderers, rapists, thieves, whores, civil-rights workers, priests; all, on the face of it, good people, until their proclivities are let loose in an access of primitive rage.

This, then, is what lies behind my sister's smiling, angelic face. Do not be fooled by the apparent innocence of the persona forced on us by civilization.

Devastating though this revelation is, it provides E—, as well as P—, with the prospect of a new and much happier life – presented to them by the Idiot they have so long denied.

I therefore withdraw all accusations and condemnations, and wish you all, with every fibre of my being, a happy and prosperous future.

THE CONTINUING LETTER TO DR G AND PSYCHIATRY

Referring to my forthcoming book, 'The Knowledge Of Everything': if you insist that ordinary human beings can possess the knowledge of everything, which is apparently the basis of your objection to me, you thereby deprive the prophet of his birthright, which quite categorically states that the prophet is distinguished from human- kind by his ability to think, which is necessary in any theory of everything; furthermore, thinking is particularly lacking in psychologists like you and Moosa, who are forced, when not abusing your patients, to spend your time abusing yourselves, either with deficiency in logic or deficiency in emotional maturity. Consequently hospitals are full of unthinking and immature doctors who are charged with the instruction of backward patients, in the art of love, with probably less knowledge than the patients themselves.

Returning to diagnosis:

It is not that these doctors <u>think</u> people are mad, but that they are <u>determined</u> to think they are mad. This is the way of <u>all</u> <u>psychological diagnosis</u>, whether you doctors are conscious of it or not. Psychiatrists, coming from their own ego, are oblivious to the truth; therefore they are unable to determine from the outset whether someone is actually mad or not. Failing this, their next step is to <u>assume</u> he is mad – because he could not possibly be otherwise, could he? Not when all my experience tells me to conclude from his mere presence in the surgery that he <u>is</u> mad, and then supply the information to prove it. Arse-ways-about thinking. But the information comes from the experience, and as we know, the experience of a psychiatric doctor is severely limited, coming, indeed, from a total <u>lack</u> of experience in the real world.

The average psychiatrist probably comes from a relatively poor background; the aristocrats don't go in for it (probably being too egotistical) and public school types, while they may be intelligent enough, generally haven't the gumption. The main run of these people, by way of their comparatively impoverished upbringing, are closer to the realities of life, and consequently have less egotism, but what they do not possess in abundance is that necessary thing, intelligence. Public schools may supply intelligence, but they also supply a persistent lack of human sympathy; the poorer grammar schools produce a mediocre type who is really not much good at anything, and really finds it hard to distinguish between a psychosis and a jelly-fish, unless one or the other stands up and says, 'This way to diagnosis', whereupon he dons his thinking cap and decides there is no difference at all – which leads him to the conclusion that all illnesses are the same, and that everyone suspected of madness automatically is so.

You will, of course, not credit this – it is in fact incredible – but having observed life as I have, from the cesspit in which I was submerged from a very early age, let me assure you that the two most prominent things in a man's life are self-love and the incapacity to think – each feeding the other. You will probably deny that the egoic processes I have described do take place, and even that they could take place; you have to know psychology to determine that, but let me point out that the undoubted susceptibilities of psychiatrists, thus exhibited, <u>exist entirely because they are unconscious of them.</u> Unconsciousness is the major fact of existence, and if it were not for that, these unfortunate people would be able to recognize, and deal with, their debilitating condition. All human beings suffer from it; psychologists are no exception, and though it must seem unbelievable that such a state of affairs could exist in the first place, it will one day be acknowledged that this extreme condition of man <u>can only be relieved by the introduction of consciousness, in order to reveal it initially and then to cure it. Consciousness was put on earth to do that.</u>

As psychologists are paid to know, but don't, unconscious darkness pervades the physical universe; we are put into the universe to learn, by the experience of life, the way to become conscious, and thus to banish darkness by thinking. Therefore thinking is important; unfortunately man has not yet developed this faculty; which is why Christ has come to teach him.

Putting Christ aside for the moment, it must be obvious by now that the physicians in charge of our welfare are very much in need of treatment themselves, as a few of the more enlightened ones will admit, but their desperate need of consciousness, which would heal them, is denied them by the very egotism which established their darkness in the first place; ego leads to non-thinking, non-thinking leads to ego. Despite the fact that the ego itself, in its natural state, is actually the area of consciousness, it becomes perverted very early on into its running-mate, egotism; the result is that the potential consciousness with which we are born, is never realized, and egotism, arising simultaneously, is determined to keep it that way. The truth being denied us, therefore, we are never able to see the psychosis threatening us.

I had written a previous letter to Dr G:

This unthinking son of India, approaching my letter with the ignorance born of his unrepentant ego, subjected it to scrutiny with his unseeing, though perceiving, eyes. On the indisputable evidence before him – the obvious fact, screaming that I could not possibly be mad – he turned away and decided that under no circumstances was he going to acknowledge it. Ignoring the logic of it – and logic unfailingly provides truth – he most illogically dismissed it. He didn't understand it, initially, because he doesn't possess reason, and he is incapable of retaining a prolonged argument in his head anyway. On this basis he condemned me as a schizophrenic.

Was this man so dense that his ego would not let him acknowledge the evidence of his own eyes? – so dense that he was not even aware that his ego was responsible? In order to accept this we have first to believe that such a thing is possible, and it is only possible when one realizes the utter shambles at the heart of the egoic experience. So great is the power of self-love that, even if we were wallowing in shit, it would convince us that we were Cleopatra. And even though this man has presumably received training, his arrant conceit still asserts itself.

Physicians refuse to accept that their diagnosis could be wrong; further, they refuse to accept even the possibility that it could be wrong. This incredible fact has to be understood in order to gain acceptance, and originates, as ever, in ego. Egotism is so fundamental to our nature that it probably covers about ninety per- cent of our negative experience, thereby rendering it impossible for us to see beyond it; spreading its tentacles throughout the whole area of the unconscious – and egotism is essentially unconscious – it suffuses every psychological function, thereby paralysing it in all but its most elementary work; an egotist is a non-functioning individual, in whom most areas of the psyche are in a parlous and immature state. Granted, most people, including psychiatrists, appear fairly mature – the schizophrenic situation (conscious versus unconscious) is the one thing above all that a psychiatrist can never afford to admit to himself – but only in irrelevant aspects, such as the ability to put two and two together or to have sexual intercourse – the two main factors in the standard test for mental aptitude; if you can prove you are good at mathematics, and equally good at getting your leg over, you are nine-tenths of the way to convincing a psychologist that you are a viable human being. Beyond that, they don't think, and it doesn't even occur to them that the one thing marking us off from animals, and the only thing that actually indicates maturity, is the very ability to think; the mathematical facility in fact indicates a total absence of thought, being based largely on a good memory (which even cockatoos have) and the capacity for ignoring logic. If you will excuse the divergence, I will amplify this. Mathematics being the least of the mental faculties, by its very nature, and particularly because of its involvement in science, is most clearly defined by its lack of logic; which is of course strange, considering the universal belief that scientists and others are such very clever fellows. In place of logic, mathematics interposes a series of assumptions based on original theories, but relying on those theories without, in the case of most mathematicians, being able to prove them; the fact that they work doesn't mean that the average scientist is responsible for them or even understands them, and pulling things out of a hat, i.e. placing blind faith in the original theorist's machinations, does not equip one for working in the real world; one only gets away with it because the world of physics is constructed around an all-inclusive, unconscious whole, in which everything is mutually supportive, and consequently it doesn't require intellectual exertion.

Logic is the first requirement of thought – bar one: intuition. Intuition is even more absent from the mathematical mind than logic, which severely restricts the likelihood of intelligence; as I have frequently pointed out, the chief distinction of the scientist is his lack of intelligence, the ability to put two and two together being a very poor substitute. Intelligence, logic, and intuition are all marked by their association with the qualities of emotion, on the one hand, and imagination on the other; without these two requirements, no function, or faculty, can be deemed competent.

The withdrawal of intuition and imagination from the field of. mathematics, which may originally have been in possession of them in the days of Pythagoras, before psychological disintegration set in, means that this discipline is now in a dysfunctional state.

The mathematician does not <u>think</u>, he is <u>thought</u>.

It is part of my procedure, when dealing with peoples' egos, to reduce the person himself to a pile of trembling shreds. Only when facing himself in the ultimate disgrace of all human nature, will man discover the truth, about himself and all men, that will give him the strength to rise up again. Wallow in the shit, therefore – in the pit of hell, indeed – and you will finally learn your own reality; what more could you want than that? This is the God-sent material on which to build your life again; taking your life in your hands, and learning to love yourself, you will emerge a new man. And you will thank me for it.

Do not imagine that my authority arises from nothing: I was there with you in that shit, eating it daily, having it forced down my throat; so nauseous was it that I lay on my back, vomiting. In this extreme, I passed most of my life, and it was only recently that I dragged myself out of it – without, I may say, any help from psychiatry, who did their best to keep me in it.

Psychiatry, my family and my own stepmother have recently conspired to deliberately re-submerge me in the death from which I have just resurrected myself, on the grounds that the life I now exhibit is indicative of mental illness. No intelligent being could deny that the reason I was forced to shout at them was the ghastly prospect before me, which I was unable to get across to them, and which consisted specifically of the re-imposition of the drugs which I had thrown off, and forcible detention in hospital – both of which have very recently been realized. (My battle in hospital has to be seen to be believed). This was the reason for what little shouting I did: what would you have done in my position? – meekly submitted? But then, these people aren't intelligent. <u>The death from which I have released myself has been the stark reality of my life almost since my birth; although I was born with a silver spoon in my mouth, that spoon was soon taken away.</u> My family might have been expected to realize my plight; but no such hope. Their only intention is to prove that everything I am saying is a lie – through their own intractable ego. They can't see it, and they are determined to prevent anyone else seeing it. They <u>know</u>, alright; but they are hell-bent on keeping it unconscious. Consciousness <u>could</u> save them, but that can only come about through their acknowledgement of my crucifixion, which they are so intent on denying.

The lifelong belief, on the part of my sister, that I am weak, is partly responsible for her failure to see the truth, and was imposed specifically to relieve her of the necessity to acknowledge it.

It is to this extent that egotism affects all men.

The vindictive repression against myself surely demonstrates the extremes to which the ego is prepared to go in defence of its unwarranted self-belief- even to denying its own God.

I bring truth, in part manifesting the boundless vitality resting within myself: the power of the universe entering me and emanating from me. This is regarded as 'manic behaviour' – even though it is entirely measured and positive. I could stop it at any time, and in any case, I choose my moments; it is never non-stop.

If you doubt the presence of God on earth, you have only to look at me.

Tidmarsh

To return to the initial diagnosis of forty years ago. I am no longer weak enough to dismiss my own conclusion that 'The rule proves the exception'; the ruling of the sitting doctor, whose name was Tidmarsh, ensues from his own egotistical incapacity to acknowledge the truth, which was evident before him. I, Anthony Wakefield Hill, was obviously not a schizophrenic, despite what I may have declared. Ignoring the facts, like every doctor since, he wilfully asserted his own self-conceit – a conceit which says, 'Under no circumstances can anyone be greater than me'; meaning that even Christ has to take a back seat. For, the quite obvious circumstances were that I had been proclaimed as Christ – not by myself – five years before, as everybody knew, and therefore he must have known that himself- particularly as I was present at the time in the very hospital where he worked. He undoubtedly knew that I had been discharged from Horton as being not only free of any mental illness but also in possession of the identity of the prophet. Argue with three psychoanalysts, plus the consultant psychiatrists, at Horton, who freed me.

Despite the evidence, then, that I was not an idiot, that I could not be considered mentally un-accountable, and that I had been declared the prophet of the age by three eminent analysts, this bespectacled son of Satan took it upon himself to ignore all this in favour of the single cry, 'Yes!' in response to the impertinent question, 'Do you hear voices?' So incensed was I by the imputation, that I decided to take the most direct route to denying it; which was to affirm it. In my book, if something is obvious, it doesn't need declaring, and the most obvious way to declare it, anyway, is to deny it. – Logic which, I am afraid, Tidmarsh and just about everybody else is incapable of comprehending.

Surely the doubt must have arisen in his mind? And, doubting it <u>unconsciously</u>, as he must have done, he <u>also unconsciously</u> proceeded to condemn Christ to a lifetime of crucifixion: as he said to me, when I asked him how long I was likely to be on the pills, 'For the rest of your life'. I retired, left to my fate.

Tidmarsh, of course, was a very nice chap – my friend, in fact – but his underlying, unconscious attitude was diabolical; as I said, in answer to the question, 'What do you think of this man?' – 'As a friend he's alright, but as a doctor he's a bastard!'

This paradoxical dichotomy is the basis of all human psychology, being founded on the schizophrenic détente between the conscious and unconscious minds which has vitiated man's affairs since Moses, and been exacerbated finally by the ever-present factor of Ego.

Why Psychiatrists Are Incapable Of Making A Diagnosis
or: Logic In Extremis

All diagnoses are descriptions, not reasons, and without a reason one hasn't proved anything. If Dr G diagnoses 'Wankers' Colic' because George's cock is as big as a tree-trunk, it merely proves that George's cock is as big as a tree-trunk, not that he is suffering from 'Wanker's Colic'. There is a distinct discrepancy here between the observed fact and the eventual analysis, which isn't an analysis at all, because it doesn't contain a reason. You can observe a chopper the size of a tree-trunk, but to apply 'Wanker's Colic' to it you would need to prove that the chopper actually earned the title; what has an inoffensive penis to do with wanking? 'Obvious', you may reply, but while penises are often used for wanking, no-one has ever proved that is their purpose. So with its purpose disproved – or rather, unproved – how can George's chopper possibly be guilty of 'Colic'? – unless Father Christmas suddenly got in and disported himself with George's own chopper – without his permission, of course – which leaves us with a very strange situation: we have, on the one hand, George being sexually abused, and on the other hand, Father Christmas behaving like a bloody schizophrenic! He doesn't know whose chopper he's holding in his hand, and the reindeer are knocking at his door, wondering when the silly old buggar is going to come out and feed them; which he won't do until he's reached his climax; and he can't do that because he doesn't know whose chopper he's holding: George's or his own. As I said, or implied, a schizophrenic scenario; and Dr G, being almost as confused as Santa, takes leave of his senses, 'takes up the cloth' and proceeds to circumcise both pricks at once: another schizophrenic situation! So now we've got two schizophrenics for the price of one.

My advice to Dr G is, go back to India, and apply for a job as the temple circumciser; that way, you won't know whether you're coming or going, and you won't be any bloody worse off – will you?

And thus subside all psychiatrists who have ever tried to make a diagnosis.

Dr L

The nonsense foisted on me by you and your side-kick has ranged from the infantile and farcical, to the most insulting and impertinent that could be conceived. You delegate your responsibilities to a drip of a schoolgirl, half my age, who barely knows one end of a condom from the other; what chance does she stand in the cockpit of life, which she has not entered, and in which I have been stationed since I was in my nappies?

What training has she had? – or you, yourself, for that matter? A South African seminar, three days a week, for four years – against fifty years in the Gulag? Gestalt and Freud only fit you for one thing: shagging and shouting; the more you shag, the more your ego is increased – and the thicker your lipstick becomes – and the louder you shout, the more you are congratulated by the 'free-thinking' fraternity – until you are brought up sharpish by the spinsters' society, who forbid any manifestation of anger – even when it is necessary.

The man who wrote the 'Knowledge Of Everything' cannot but be the Prophet: no ordinary human being could possibly be in possession of the knowledge of everything – unless you consider that this is not a knowledge of everything, in other words a hoax, or that the writer of the report is a liar, or that I am a liar myself in claiming to be the author. If you insist on asserting these things, you are dismissing logic, reason and proof, and only proving, in fact, that you are not competent to be a psychiatrist.

It is the rule that proves the exception, Christ being the only man in step.

You are obviously determined, right from the start, not to believe that <u>it is even possible</u> for someone to be Christ. That is the sole basis for your argument; in fact, you haven't an argument: you are just blind assertion.

I have yet to hear one coherent reason for psychiatry's denial that I am Christ – apart from the fact that it is highly unlikely –

something which I fully endorse, no-one being more surprised than I am. That, indeed, is why I am ill. An identity crisis, you see.

For sixty-four years, I have been pursuing a course of equally blind denial: the denial of my own identity. I can deny it no longer; if I don't come out now, the world will be left to its fate.

I am going to be crucified, again, in the not-too distant future – in a particularly horrible and gruesome manner – far worse than crucifixion on a cross. I am going into this willingly and consciously, because if I don't, it will never happen, and if it doesn't happen, you, and women like you, will never have your pants taken off again – for the simple reason that there will be no men left to take them off, all of them losing their lives in the very probable nuclear conflagration.

Only I can prevent this.

I take a high tone with everyone; that is my approach. I lay down the law because I am the authority, and I do not expect any impertinent comeback from anybody.

I have spent the last sixty years of my life in anonymity, because of my own self-disbelief, but I am now asserting who I am. I will do this in no uncertain manner, as it is only by thrusting man's recalcitrance down his own throat that I will stand any chance of being accepted in a world that actually belongs to me. 'Gentle Jesus, meek and mild', is a thing of the past, not having any relevance today. Take the buggers by storm, I say.

If it is your intention to prosecute me, I would be delighted – but do read my essay properly, first.

I hereby declare

that I am Christ,

and that I intend to

shout at everyone

in the universe –

with the express intention

of being intimidating;

until they have

heard my Word

Christmas Eve at Gale Cottage

My father was an infrequent visitor to Gale Cottage, mainly because the bloody place was so cold! There was no central-heating, and the bedrooms were absolutely freezing; as my Uncle, another infrequent visitor, said, 'Getting out of bed for a piss was an act of great bravery' – which may have been why my Grandmother frequently pissed the bed – though that was aggravated by her over-fondness for the gin-bottle. Her eagerness in this regard communicated itself, on most Christmas Eves, to the guests, among whom was the Inspector of Police, who was so plied with drink that he once climbed into his car backwards, and attempted to manipulate the steering-wheel with his arse (no mean feat).

One particular Christmas, during the war, my Father returned from North Africa – with a mission. Now, to put it mildly, he and my Grandmother did not get on, and although he had tried to get rid of her on several occasions, once with poison, once by attempting to strangle her with my Mother's tights, the old girl wouldn't die; and during the whole of his sojourn in North Africa – where he became the only man to be decorated by Monty for his service in the desert latrines (apparently Rommel stumbled into the camp one night after a drunken bout, and proceeded to have a crap, whereupon my Father, who had nerves of steel, placed him under shit-house arrest) – he became obsessed by the desire to liquidate this rabid old woman. I never did find out exactly why he conceived such a hatred for her; perhaps it was because she used to fart like a trooper – God rest her soul – which was enough to put anyone off his dinner. However, this Christmas he was determined to deliver the coup-de- grace, so, one day when the old girl wandered down to the privy, at the bottom of the garden, he sneaked up and lobbed a hand- grenade in. There was a tremendous explosion. Then, suddenly, my Grandmother came rushing out yelling, 'The pills have worked! The pills have worked!'

You can imagine my Father's disappointment – the poor bugger had failed again! Of course, when my Mother found out, she immediately 'stopped his cock', as they say; which was a worse punishment, as far as he was concerned, than being hanged.

Well, in time, of course, the happy family settled down again, and things pursued their humdrum course until the next Christmas, when Father dressed up, as usual, as Santa. Now, it so happened that the previous year, during all the carousing, I was ensconced in bed, enthusiastically addressing my foreskin, when Father, dressed as Santa, emerged from the chimney: 'You dirty little buggar!' he exclaimed, and proceeded to thrash me. Well, as you can imagine, I was mortified, and I determined to teach him a lesson; so, the next year, I decided to catch the old bastard coming down the chimney, as he usually did. I laid my plans carefully, and as soon as I heard him come back from the pub – I was alerted by a stentorian fart from the cook, to which my Father replied, quite audibly, 'Thanks, Ivy!' – I tiptoed into Ivy's bedroom and commandeered her pisspot, plus a bit of elastic which I extracted from her outsize bloomers. Now, I reckoned that, if all went according to plan, Father would start down the chimney dead on the stroke of midnight, so I stretched the elastic right across the front of the chimney, with the Po strategically placed in line with it. Well, sure enough, as the clock struck twelve, Wing-Commander W.O. Hill descended the chimney, and I was not disappointed at the result. As soon as he stepped out of the chimney-breast, he tripped over the elastic, and landed face-first in the piss-pot. My cup of happiness, also, brimmed over!

My days at Gale were tolerably happy, but they came to an abrupt end when I was summarily dispatched to a distant boarding school. It came about in this way: I was a pupil at the local primary school, and as I was a shy sort of chap, Mary, who, as you know, was a teacher at the same school, introduced me to a certain girl, who Mary hoped would befriend me and 'show me the ropes'. Well, she did show me the ropes – in no uncertain manner – in fact she 'showed' me more than the ropes! Although I was unable to perform to her satisfaction (being only five or six years old) this little minx did the dirty on me, and when I got home that night, my Father was waiting for me. 'What do you mean by shagging the Group Captain's daughter, you little horror?' Well, I was perplexed; I had no idea what 'sex' was, let alone that I had actually performed it. But this girl had informed my sister that I was the instigator, and my sister, who hated me cordially, was delighted at the chance to get me into trouble. So I decided to get my own back. Quite soon after the above event, my sister was laid up in bed, so I got an old lemonade bottle, pissed in it, and gave it to her to drink. Needless to say, I did a hasty bunk before anything happened, but, of course, my mother was irate, and wasted no time in expelling me from the happy home. (Unfortunately, history does not record whether or not my sister actually drank the 'beverage', a matter which has consumed me with curiosity ever since).

However, all's well that ends well, and though I can't relate that either my Father or my Grandmother are yet dead, I can tell you that Pom Boustead, the gardener, who as you know was addicted to methylated spirits, promoted himself in my eyes by having the temerity to betake himself, that Christmas, to my Mother's bed – boots on and all! (Of course, my Mother wasn't there at the time, being busy with my Grandmother downstairs at the gin bottle). But what made my day was that Ivy – the fat cow – discovered Boustead in Mama's bed, and much to my delight, the drunken gardener, on being roused from his slumbers, proceeded to exhibit his outsize genitalia to the astonished cook, who took one look and promptly fled. I should explain that Boustead, who had recently attempted to 'plight his troth' with Ivy, had been rejected – largely because the unfortunate woman was 'thimble-twatted' and couldn't admit a man to her trysting-place – even supposing you could find it, she was so fat. As Freud would say, this was obviously a case of frustration on the part of the gardener and sour grapes on the part of the cook, who wasted no time in reporting the matter to my Grandfather. Now, being a Quaker, my Grandfather was doubly incensed at the gardener's lapse, and after docking his pay for a week, he sent him to see the vicar, who really read him the riot-act: 'Thou shalt not exhibit thy genitals in public', (saith the Lord). But I am happy to report that my good friend, Boustead, was so shocked by the vicar's response that he swore never to touch another drop of drink – and from that day to this, he hasn't!

The Department of Continuous Clinical Improvement has been shaken to its foundations by rumours of a sinister underground society, operating within an organization which I cannot name for legal reasons. The secret society calls itself the Brotherhood of the Blanket, with obvious allusions to the ancient order founded by the 6th century mystic, Dionysius the Pseudo-Aeropagite. This former hamburger magnate underwent a dramatic conversion experience, and promptly eschewed the fast food trade to found a charitable Order of Hospitallers. They conveniently disappeared from the history books to escape dissolution by Henry VIII – until now.

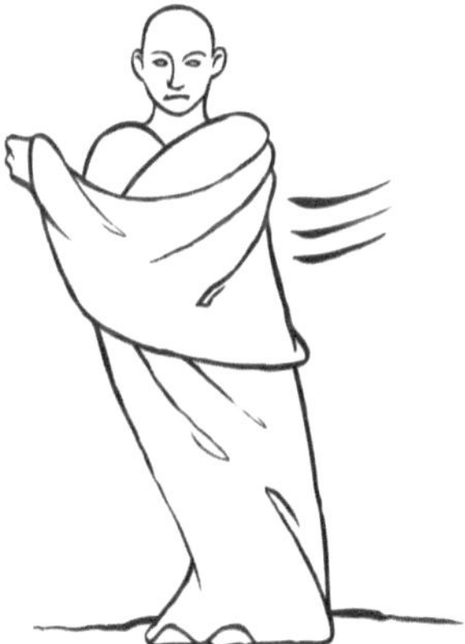

As yet, little is known about the Brotherhood. They may well have financed the construction of Hillview Hospital, so that the Deserving Poor could receive primitive medical help and the cure of souls. The original Brotherhood were evidently dedicated to the less fortunate. Further investigation is needed to determine whether Christian Hospitality is the true purpose of their modern counter-parts, or merely a front for some mysterious unmentionable activity. The way they appear to glide up and down the wards at an uncanny speed, with blankets billowing out behind them, certainly demands an explanation…

164

*To Mr James Warburton of the Emporium Wine
Bar and his manageress, having been chucked out.*

A mistake has been made. You, obviously, are unaware of what
ensued. And I do not take kindly to the distasteful accusation,
from an impertinent young girl like you, that I would even
contemplate discussing a woman's knickers with her. I have a
damned good mind to take you to court and make your face go
red – if it's capable of it.

In the first place, there was not one girl involved, but two, and
this schizophrenic confusion evidently results from the fact that
you received your information from a third party, in a garbled
manner. If you are going to accuse me, at least make sure of your
facts, and if there is any suggestion of an attempt to charm the
girl's pants off her, I require material evidence; the said pants will
need to be presented in court – otherwise I disclaim any such
design.

This whole business started when I sat down in the
Emporium and waited to be served; I waited at least ten minutes
without anyone approaching me, all the waitresses passing to and
fro in front of me without bestowing a glance, even attending
people who had walked in after me; as usual, I seem to be
invisible, though the position of that chair does not demand its
dismissal from consciousness. When this male waiter walked past,
also ignoring me, I hailed him, emphatically saying, 'Can I have
some service?' – a normal thing in my opinion. I was surprised at
the time that he didn't assert his amour-propre, but he reserved
this for the later event. When I had delivered my order, my
annoyance subsided and as far as I was concerned that was the end
of the matter.

Just as I finished my meal, the waitress in question, with
whom I was on very friendly terms, appeared in the offing.
Thinking she was receptive to a humorous approach, I essayed a

joke in her direction, which did not concern <u>her</u> underwear at all. This is what I said, 'Have you got a spare pair of underpants (meaning men's underpants) because I can't find any to fit me?' – Is she likely to have a pair of men's underpants in her pocket? It is so unlikely that it formed the first part of the joke. I immediately went on to the main point of the joke, 'Has your boyfriend got a spare pair?' <u>Obviously indicating it was not her underwear I was talking about.</u> I have been unable to find a pair of underpants to fit me for a long time, and this has formed a subject of amusement on many occasions with other girls – including Tara – who have invariably received it humorously. The idea that I was intending to swap our underwear is ludicrous; how could I possibly expect to wear a pair of women's pants? And I didn't make any unseemly allusions whatever to female undergarments. I am not in the habit of making 'obscene' or 'offensive' remarks to any woman, whatever age she is.

The whole thing is nonsense and was intended to be nonsense, by me, from the start; it could only have been regarded as a joke – that was patently obvious. This girl must have been surpassingly stupid.

I later went upstairs to say goodbye to my special friend, Tara, who had told me she was leaving. I wanted to make sure she knew how much I loved her (and how much she loved me, incidentally) in a few short words because I knew she was busy. My opening shot was, 'How can I make love to you before Monday?' – the day she was leaving. She was very well aware that, being the person I am, I have never made love to any woman, nor have I any intention of ever doing so; therefore such a 'threat' was empty and was only intended to convey my very honourable feelings – as a totally disinterested send-off. I would never have seen her again and I very nearly didn't bother going up there in the first place. I am who I am, and I do this for all females everywhere – without hope of return.

Tara protested that she had a boyfriend; I knew this perfectly well, and precisely because I have never done such a thing, I said, 'I eat boyfriends for breakfast!' This was absolutely untrue, and my sole object was to prove my overwhelming love for this girl in as forceful and unmistakable manner as I could. It did, of course, fall flat.

Knowing that I could not let the situation rest there, I immediately followed it up, as she turned to go into the kitchen, with the words, 'One day you will see that I have every right to take any woman I want.' It is perfectly true that I have this right, as everyone will see before long, but in fact I have never availed myself of the right and have no desire to do so; I would regard it as a mortal sin.

On this basis, therefore, anyone with intelligence can see that my behaviour towards Tara did not warrant my being chucked out, and I cannot be held responsible for her failure to see the truth. For Tara's relationship with me needs to be understood. She and I were deeply in love for many months, but it was she who first approached me, despite what you may think. Of all the stupid flibbertigibbets in the Emporium, only Tara drew my real attention; I told her: 'Although I may be in love with all these other girls you are the only one I would seriously consider doing.' That went straight to her heart and her lovely little body at the same time; and from then on she was mine, despite the fact that I probably would never have done anybody at all – as she knew, because I had previously told her that I was not allowed to consort with women, due to my religion.

Being very much in love with me, then, Tara continued for some time, but when it became clear that neither of us were going to realise our dreams, she became very unhappy. I am almost certain that she had never had a boyfriend – she was such an exquisite, exceptional creature – and when the one man in her life proved to be unrealisable, she was forced to give up hope and thrust me underground. She proceeded from then on almost entirely unconscious of me, sometimes being virtually hostile when I appeared in front of her. Knowing that her feelings were, however, exactly the opposite, I never failed to assure her of my love, which, despite herself she accepted; this assiduous devotion was, I believe, regarded as 'stalking' by some of the other unintelligent little smellies. But I was determined not to let her go unnourished, knowing, of course, that there was no hope for me either, and in my earthly guise as the 'idiot' I pursued her about with endless jokes, which were usually welcomed – the more explicit and daring the better, and these were never rejected by a girl who, though so young, was so mature and womanly.

She eventually took up with some kind of boyfriend, reluctantly, which I was glad to hear for her sake, and I never attempted to dislodge her from him – knowing however that she did not love him and he was incapable of loving her. Once again I saw the girl I loved go to an undeserving poltroon.

This was the situation when, for whatever reason, she announced she was leaving. Gobsmacked, I had to let her go. I will not be accused of degrading Tara.

Enter the waiter. Being a person moved exclusively by his own ego – which shouted itself by his long nose – he unfailingly took umbrage at my original demand for service, which made him look slightly small and, upstairs in the bar, it came out. I had not 'raised my voice' in any way whatever – I don't usually do that kind of thing unless it is justified and under exceptional circumstances – until Tara turned to go into the kitchen, upon which, because there was such a din in the place, I was forced to do so a very slight extent – no more. It did not merit the reaction it got; the waiter, seeing his opportunity, immediately jumped in (with raised voice) demanding, 'Calm down, sir, or I'll have to ask you to leave!' He had the perfect excuse, though this was not of course the reason. Having observed egotism all my life, and long noses, this was what I expected. To start with there was no need to tell me to 'calm down' because I was not 'worked up', as he knew; nor did I exhibit any trace of anger or any other obstreperous emotion. To order me out on such a pretext, quite apart from its enormity, illustrates the disastrous influence of egotistical conviction on the psyche of man in general. This was exacerbated in his case when he heard my declaration to Tara; his masculinity was offended by the temerity of another male in demonstrating his superior ability with women on his territory. Down, as ever, comes the hatchet. And as everyone else's pride was immediately injured for the same reason, I received universal condemnation, which the witnesses presented to you as a demand for my expulsion.

I do not know what Tara may or may not have told you, but you must realise that women in such a situation are likely to say the opposite of what their feelings actually are for the man engaging their affections. The more they can hurt him, the better. And under the circumstances, Tara was also, understandably, confused; she was not offended by what I said, but simply taken aback by the truth it revealed about her real emotions. So she came out, I have no doubt, spitting and snarling. This reaction – which I deliberately provoked and desired – is the preliminary to her awakening, and will be healed when she eventually realises who I am. This is my procedure in most cases of emotional crisis; the 'patient' has to be reduced by shock to a state of receptivity to the truth, which is in most cases very unwelcome; what we are hiding from ourselves is always devastating when first presented to consciousness, but it is this very conscious presentation which, almost by itself, provides the cure. Grasping the unpalatable truth, we can either affirm it or deny it, depending upon which we are enabled to proceed into the New Life, which I hold out to every man and woman. In Tara's case the truth is my identity.

No, I am not a witch-doctor – no I am not mad; and that much vilified 'Journal' would prove it to anyone intelligent enough to give it a chance.

That was the best parting gift I could have given Tara.

Your immediate response as a professional provocateuse, incapable of thought, will be: 'We are not prepared to listen to your argument – you have offended two members of our staff and that is that. Two little skivvies carry much more weight than you – the more lies they tell, the better. We are not moved by reason – such a thing would not enter our heads – and Mr Warburton is well-known to defend the weak against all truth – his charitable instincts persuading him to expel all exponents of that quality.'

In this country you do not hang a man for murder without knowing his motives: it is regarded as a gross injustice and contrary to the laws of logic, everywhere but in the Emporium. That fact that you do not like me, and are offended by any evidence of reality, does not provide you with sufficient justification to get rid of me. But no doubt you will, guided solely by the dictates of outraged propriety; and once again the representative of Innocence itself falls a victim, martyred to a pair of stinking knickers.

I find it in the highest degree offensive that I should have been ejected from the Emporium without any justifiable reason, but purely on the grounds of a waiter's egotism and the susceptibilities of a couple of silly school girls.

I have no reason to accuse myself of anything distasteful, and indeed if your idea of underpants conjures up a dirty image, the dirtiness is in your mind, not mine. Perhaps you should wash yours more often.

Christ's message is, as ever: do not judge by appearances – the truth will escape you.

In a few months' time, the identity of the man you have thus abused, will be revealed to the world at large.

Anthony Wakefield Hill

Appendix

P.92 – I wish to avert the dilemma entailed in the statement that I was admitted to hospital on physical grounds, not mental. What I meant was that I have never been mentally ill, therefore never genuinely on mental grounds.